The International Behavioural and Social Sciences Library

IDENTITY

TAVISTOCK

The International Behavioural and Social Sciences Library

PSYCHOLOGY
In 11 Volumes

I	Current Trends in Analytical Psychology
	Edited by Gerhard Adler
II	Focal Psychotherapy
	Michael Balint, et al.
III	Primary Love and Psycho-Analytic Technique
	Michael Balint
IV	Attention and Interpretation
	W R Bion
V	Themes in Speculative Psychology
	Nehemiah Jordan
VI	Envy and Gratitude
	Melanie Klein
VII	New Directions in Psycho-Analysis
	Edited by Melanie Klein, et al.
VIII	A Study of Brief Psychotherapy
	D H Malan
IX	Displacement of Concepts
	Donald A Schon
X	Identity
	Edited by Kenneth Soddy
XI	System and Structure
	Anthony Wilden

IDENTITY

Mental Health and Value Systems

EDITED BY KENNETH SODDY

First published in 1961 by
Tavistock Publications (1959) Limited

Reprinted in 2001 by
Routledge
2 Park Square, Milton Park, Abingdon, Oxon, OX14 4RN

Transferred to Digital Printing 2007

Routledge is an imprint of the Taylor & Francis Group

© 1961 World Federation for Mental Health

British Library Cataloguing in Publication Data
A CIP catalogue record for this book
is available from the British Library

Identity
ISBN 0-415-26487-1
Psychology: 11 Volumes
ISBN 0-415-26515-0
The International Behavioural and Social Sciences Library
112 Volumes
ISBN 0-415-25670-4

CROSS-CULTURAL STUDIES IN
MENTAL HEALTH

Identity

*

Mental Health and Value Systems

EDITOR
KENNETH SODDY

TAVISTOCK PUBLICATIONS

First published in 1961
by Tavistock Publications (1959) Limited
2 Park Square, Milton Park, Abingdon, Oxon, OX14 4RN
in 11/12 point Baskerville
by Staples Printers Limited at their
Rochester, Kent, establishment

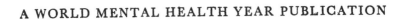

A WORLD MENTAL HEALTH YEAR PUBLICATION

WORLD FEDERATION FOR MENTAL HEALTH

FÉDÉRATION MONDIALE POUR LA SANTÉ MENTALE

CONTENTS

PREFACE   xi

ACKNOWLEDGEMENTS   xii

Identity

INTRODUCTION   I
*Reason for working – Reason for choosing 'identity'
– References to identity*

I.   DEFINITIONS   3

II. FIRST APPROACH TO IDENTITY   4
     Reciprocity – Continuum

III. THE DEVELOPMENT OF IDENTITY   5
     *Twins – The course of development – somatic sensi-
     tivity – Identity organization – Time scale of ego and
     identity formation*

IV. EMPATHY   9
     *Sex differences in empathy formation – Empathy
     and burial or cremation wishes*

V.   IDENTIFICATION WITH OTHERS   I2
     *Child-parent identification – Friendship, courtship,
     and mating – Hatred and identification – Extreme
     emphasis on identity factors*

VI. IDENTITY AND GROUP MEMBERSHIP   I5
     *Group loyalties – Group prejudice – Laughter –
     Roots – Leadership – In-groups and out-groups
     – Reference groups – Morality – Identity change
     – Individuality and group – Individualism and
     collectivism*

vii

VII. FURTHER ASPECTS OF IDENTIFICATION   25
     How are individuals identified? – Labels – Identi-
     fication in families – Identity as an interpersonal
     phenomenon

VIII. FURTHER CULTURAL FACTORS AND IDENTITY   30
     Social role, status, and class – Some peer culture
     phenomena – Nationalism

IX. IDENTITY CONTINUITY, COHERENCE, AND FLEXIBILITY   34
     Some ethnological considerations – Personality inte-
     gration – Identity strength – Formalized ways of
     accepting temporary breaks in identity – Promotion
     of identity strength – Prevention of excessive strain
     on identity formation

X. HIERARCHY OF IDENTITIES   38
     Multiple identities – Hierarchy of identities – Basic
     plot – Style of identity

XI. UNUSUAL FORMS OF IDENTITY   42
     Change of identity – Migration – 'Family romance'

XII. MORE EXTREME FORMS OF IDENTITY FORMATION   45
     Social conventions permitting changes of identity
     – Specific sources of strain – Special position of some
     individuals and whole groups – Double personality –
     Disturbances of identity

XIII. IDENTITY BREAKDOWN   48
     Depersonalization – Attitudes to death

XIV. MENTAL HEALTH IMPLICATIONS   50

     REFERENCES   52

Mental Health and Value Systems

EDITORIAL NOTE   57

INTRODUCTION   59

Background to this study – The selection of the subject – The general aim – Cross-cultural application – The range of the problems – The measurement of mental health

1. MENTAL HEALTH ASSUMPTIONS AND IMPLICATIONS   70

The nature of mental health – Deviant behaviour – Social relationships – Universal phenomena – Summary

2. RELEVANT MATERIAL FROM VARIOUS RELIGIONS AND IDEOLOGIES   118

Introduction – Variations in value systems – Responsibility – Identity – Flexibility – Social organization – Concepts of right and wrong – Different attitudes to suffering, death, guilt – Attitudes towards mental illness – Similarities – Summary

3. SOME PRACTICAL IMPLICATIONS   169

Some specific conditions affecting mental health work – Some more theoretical considerations – Summary

4. SOME LEADS INTO RESEARCH   212

Human development – Studies in psychology and religion – Mental health practices – Further research areas

EPILOGUE   238

REFERENCES   241

RÉSUMÉ   243

RESUMEN   252

INDEXES   263

PREFACE

THE TWO studies which comprise this volume, *Identity* and *Mental Health and Value Systems*, constitute the first two Cross-Cultural Studies in Mental Health produced by the Scientific Committee of the World Federation for Mental Health. Chronologically, *Identity* appeared first, being published privately in 1957, but since it had only a very narrow circulation the opportunity has been taken to re-publish it with its successor. The Committee has varied slightly in composition between the two studies. For *Mental Health and Value Systems*, the Committee has been joined by Dr. David Levy, Professor E. F. O'Doherty, and Professor Paul Sivadon. Unfortunately Professor D. Lagache has been unable to take part in the latter study and Professor W. Line has been able to participate only by correspondence.

ACKNOWLEDGEMENTS

THE SCIENTIFIC COMMITTEE of the World Federation for Mental Health gratefully acknowledges a grant from the Edward W. Hazen Foundation, without which its study on *Mental Health and Value Systems* would not have been possible. This grant enabled us to hold conferences in New York and London respectively, which supplied the Committee with much of the material on which it has worked. We are also deeply indebted to the Council for International Organizations of Medical Sciences for a grant which made it possible for the Scientific Committee to meet at the most crucial phase of the task of compiling the report. It is largely through the generosity of these two organizations that we have been able to make our contribution to World Mental Health Year.

Identity

Identity

INTRODUCTION

IN SELECTING subjects for discussion and report, the Scientific Committee of the World Federation for Mental Health has had three possible objectives in mind:

1. To seek clarification and, if possible, consensus in an international and interprofessional sense on the more frequently used concepts in the field of mental health;

2. To review those concepts which appear to be emerging and gaining in importance;

3. To draw attention to those areas patently requiring further study.

The Scientific Committee's Report on 'Identity' is intended as the first of a series of introductory studies, from an international and interdisciplinary point of view, of basic concepts used in Mental Hygiene. It has been designed to stimulate thought and discussion, but not as an attempt to exhaust the subject. The Report is the joint work of the members of the Committee, but unfortunately Professor Lagache has been able to participate only by correspondence; and Professor Line partly by correspondence, being present in person at one of the three meetings at which the Report was discussed. In addition, the members of the Scientific Committee are greatly indebted to the many people with whom they have individually and in groups discussed the concepts underlying the Report; and particularly to the following members of the Executive Board and their colleagues who so

Identity

kindly responded to the Scientific Committee's request for comments: Dr. Estefania Aldaba-Lim (Philippines); Dr. Irene Cheng (Hong Kong); Dr. Carl Haffter (Switzerland); Professor Dr. A. C. Pacheco e Silva (Brazil); Dr. J. R. Rees (Director, WFMH); Dr. G. S. Stevenson (U.S.A); and Dr. P. M. Yap (Hong Kong).

Reason for Working

It may be asked why the Scientific Committee of the Federation is undertaking work of this kind. It is legitimate to argue that the main preoccupation of the WFMH should be with social action – with getting things improved, but in accepting this role the Federation has always been conscious of the slender conceptual foundations of most of its work. Hence the formation of the Scientific Committee, which is concerned with the attempt to develop a body of knowledge and to prepare personnel ready for action when opportunity offers; and more than this – ready to create the opportunity for appropriate action. We have a unique opportunity for coming together, from various cultures and professions, to discuss matters of mutual interest. Our ambition, like that of many other people in this field, is to do more than can be achieved by methods of survey in the field or of literature, but in the actual work represented by this document we are undertaking very much less than a survey. However, out of the material which we hope to collate, we are attempting to bring into focus and due perspective some of the current thinking on the problem of identity. In this way we hope to be able to make a positive contribution to current thought.

Reason for Choosing 'Identity'

Originally, the Committee approached its tasks through the consideration of such concepts as positive mental health, and it was found that discussion in this area almost inevitably led into the discussion of some aspect of identity. This subject, besides holding a wealth of interest of itself, seemed to be particularly relevant to the problems of the World Federation for Mental Health; concerned in principle with world citizenship, and in the practical sphere with, among other things, all the difficulties and

2

perplexities arising out of programmes of technical assistance, changing technology, population movement, and change of class. Identity is, therefore, a frequently used concept, but it is also an emerging idea.

References to Identity

Among the vast literature in this field, we would draw attention to books by Gardner Murphy (1947) and George Mead (1934) on the subject of the self, to papers by Joseph Bram and also Erik Erikson, and especially to the latter's paper on the problem of ego-identity (1956). There are many other references and not only in the psychological world. For example, Erikson has also contributed, at the 1950 White House Conference, a paper on *Search for Identity in Adolescence*. W. B. Yeats, from a more poetical angle, has written on self and anti-self. Hartley (1946) has written on children's ethnic identification, and James Plant on *Whoness and Whatness*. We would draw attention to Riesman's *Faces in the Crowd* (1952). We must not overlook the seventeenth-century writings of John Donne. Naturally, it is recognized that interest in this subject is not limited to the sciences of human behaviour. The recent popular cults of existentialism, for example, have aroused wide interest in the subject, but it is true in a more strictly scientific sense that identity is still an emerging concept. Since it also obviously includes vast areas requiring further study, it can be said, as a subject, to combine within itself all the Committee's self-appointed criteria.

I. DEFINITIONS

The Committee discussed the question of attempting to define the term identity and the related terms – ego, self, identification, individuation, individuality, personality, persona, person, character, temperament, empathy, identity strength, and ego strength. After quite prolonged discussion, which was for the members of the Committee a most illuminating and educative experience, a unified convention of use could not be found for any one of these terms. There are strong reasons for refraining from attempting a definition at the outset, indeed to succeed would beg the issue of the whole discussion.

The term 'identity' will be used in a group, as well as an individual sense, recognizing the interdependence of group and individual. The identity of an individual is a property which is inalienable from him, but in another sense, an individual's identity is only needed and, it might be argued, only *possible,* when he is a member of a group. Identity discs or tags are used not so much to define the individual, but to mark him off and separate him from all other individuals. It is implicit that a contribution to George being George is the fact that John is John. The term 'identity' will not be used in its literal derivative sense of 'absolute sameness' (Latin *idem*=same, see *Concise Oxford Dictionary*), but in the alternative meanings of 'personality' and 'individuality'.

A useful positive comment can be taken from Kluckhohn & Murray (1949) that every individual, concurrently, is, in certain respects, like all other men, some other men, and no other man. We could go further and say that this truth applies to all living beings.

II. FIRST APPROACH TO IDENTITY

Reciprocity

As a starting-point the Committee took the concept that identity is a quality or complex of qualities that an individual presents to others, but this concept leaves out of account the reciprocal nature of identity. Identity has been described more figuratively as an anchorage of the self in the social matrix, but this likewise does not give a full impression of the reciprocity of the relationship, though it shows that both aspects, the matrix and the self, are necessary.

Continuum

It will be helpful here to anticipate some of the later discussion, by way of illustration: identity is conceived of as a continuum and its loss is not an all-or-none phenomenon. That well-known war-time difficulty of soldiers' 'loss of memory' involved a partial loss or diminuation of identity without its total disappearance. In many respects the soldier would continue to carry on his ordinary duties, though he might not know his name, who, what, or where he was.

We have referred to identity as a continuum, and its loss, as in the case of the soldier, is not an all-or-none phenomenon. From the progressive loss of qualities of identity by an individual, it might be possible to grade the importance of these parts in a kind of hierarchy either in terms of individual or cultural differences (see also *Hierarchy of Identities,* pp. 38–40). For example, the loss of the proper name, so common among soldiers suffering from 'loss of memory', might occur only in those cases in which the name is a main symbol of identity. (*Note:* Loss of proper name is only one possible manifestation of loss of identity.)

Loss of memory, which will be considered again later, has other interesting aspects in that it may include a resistance to being identified. This resistance might be a possible basis of the patient's amnesia, but there are probably many other complicating factors.

It can also be mentioned that identity can be studied in terms of where the individual thinks he is going, or perhaps fears he might be going; this leads on to a speculation on the relative strengths of drives towards a goal and avoiding a foreseen end.

III. THE DEVELOPMENT OF IDENTITY

According to one of the schools of dynamic psychology, identification arises by a process of introjection or introception. We propose to use the terms introjection, incorporation, and introception as if they were more or less synonymous, but in that order implying an increasing degree of harmoniousness of the process. Identification is one of the earliest and least differentiated steps in the process of identity development, i.e. one of the ways in which an individual attains identity.

Twins

Twins show interesting aspects of identity development. Radcliffe-Brown, studying African tribes, has described how identical twins

can be regarded as an insult to the social order and their existence may arouse primitive feelings of hostility in the tribe. Twins
often have the feeling that others do not distinguish between
them and this may be a source of either satisfaction or frustration
to them.

Identity necessarily involves a differentiation of the individual
from the rest of the world, so that identical twins with an insep-
arable alter-ego will have one facet of their identity blurred.
Some twins are dependent on this alter-ego for effective functioning. The same can sometimes been seen in siblings of the same
sex and almost the same age, if brought up together and sharing
the same environment, e.g. being in the same class, experiencing
a similar psychological make-up as described in the case of twins.
The younger one is apt to identify himself or herself with the
elder one and to 'live in symbiosis' with the other one. Being
dressed in similar clothing, being mistaken for the other, etc., will
add to the feeling of 'identity'.

Sometimes the weaker twin or younger sibling does not
develop full maturity until circumstances separate him or her
from the counterpart.

Other people, who are not twins, may need to have a fantasy
twin if they cannot bear the aloneness of a separate identity.
There are many examples of the less skilful of twins living in
symbiosis with the twin as a necessary condition of the latter
functioning at his optimum level. A Belgian study in 1929
showed that in a competitive situation non-identical twins tended
to compete and identical twins to combine. This might suggest
that in some societies binovular twins are regarded as complete
entities respectively, but each of identical twins as incomplete.

However, differences may appear in identical twins brought
up together up to adulthood and then separated. A case was
quoted of two French-Canadian soldiers who during the war
served in Europe, one returned to live in France, married a
French woman, and settled there, and the other did not.

The Course of Development – Somatic Sensitivity
The phenomenon of empathy will be considered more fully at the

III. The Development of Identity

beginning of Section IV. Empathy is one of the key phenomena in the process of identification, and is therefore highly germane to identity formation. It can be defined, broadly speaking, as the capacity to feel into another; and it can be aptly illustrated by a Russian peasant saying that a woman knows that her child is hungry because her breasts hurt. (See also Sarbin, 1954, on Role Theory.)

We shall now consider some of the early steps by which empathy arises. The child's normal process of developing identity is through the sensori-motor activities of the first two years of life, which activities also are involved in the process of identification. By a ceaseless exploration a kind of somatic sensitivity develops between the child and his immediate surroundings. This somatic sensitivity is one of the roots of empathy. It may depend on a sensori-motor congruity between mother and child, and when this exists, the child is in a state of 'blessedness'. This maternal capacity is almost certainly linked with the female sex and in some cases the reaction is specific to the function of motherhood, as can be seen by the baby's differentiated response to the person who is exercising that function. The father who is taking care of his own baby might show something of the same congruity, but, possibly, this is to do with a protective rather than a nourishing function.

One of the results of somatic sensitivity is the intuitive recognition of structures and forces within the environment. A child comes to recognize intuitively such matters as, for example, gravity, or the effect of throwing a hard object across the room and hitting his mother, and thus will come to foresee intuitively the probable reaction of his mother. This might be regarded as a process of value differentiation. Then, as the process becomes more abstract, the child may reach an understanding of his own attitudes and those of others, an understanding that, at this early period, is peculiarly dependent upon the sensori-motor activities of young children. It should be remembered that, in the case of very young children, cognitive deprivation may follow upon sensori-motor restriction or disability.

In certain cases, development of somatic sensitivity may be

7

incomplete and a state may arise in which the child will put more and more exploratory motor gestures into the environment; these fail to find their objective, become repetitive and inappropriate, and serious perseveration will appear. This is an abnormal development, with serious consequences, but there remains a possibility, in some cases, that the child may later find some alternative route towards identity formation. In normal development, though empathy and identity formation acquire a slight cognitive component even as early as six months, throughout the nursery years of childhood, body learning and intuitive experiences remain the most important for the child. At the age of five or six years, new means of communion become available to the child through the rapid intellectual development that occurs at this time. Cultural patterning is significant in the timing of these processes.

In these cases of incomplete somatic sensitivity that have been mentioned, it may be found, round about the age of six, that the child may develop something of the normal child's capacity and will fill in some of the missing links of his somatic understanding, by perception and conception. Such a child will literally learn how to behave, but he will do this without a full range of feeling, intuition, or understanding. It has been noted that identity formation includes the separation of the rest of the world from the self, and so involves the acquisition of a concept of the world as well as of the self. Therefore these children will be not only deficient in their own identity formation, but they will add to this the mis-identification of objects around them. Many examples can be found of this phenomenon, of which that of Monique is the best known. (See Soddy, 1955, *Mental Health and Infant Development*, Vol. I, pp. 125–130.)

Identity Organization

An important aspect of identity organization is its degree of resistance to vicissitudes. It has often been stated that the first principle is the building up of identity strength as a positive system and not as a matter of negative identities or negative images. However, it will be better not to use a structural metaphor of 'building', but to regard this as a system of energy and to think in terms of organization, direction, and control.

A distinction needs to be made between identity strength and ego strength. Under some circumstances these may be antithetical. Ego strength is an energy-phenomenon and it includes the strength to organize experience. A strong identity may, conceivably, result in weak ego, and this will also be true of strong identification with someone else. Another antithetical ego function may be the abolition of self as in sleep, so that energy may be conserved; sleep also seriously weakens the inward aspect of identity. Another ego function is that of relating the inner world with the outer, creatively. The examples given will illustrate the need to examine still further the differentiation between the two concepts, but here we shall stop with the observation that generally identity strength and ego strength will not correspond. (See also: *Personality Integration*, p. 35; *Identity Strength*, p. 36; *Multiple Identities*, p. 38; *Hierarchy of Identities*, p. 39; *Basic Plot*, p. 40; *Style of Identity*, p. 41, in which also the question of authenticity or genuineness of individuals is discussed.)

Time Scale of Ego and Identity Formation

It is possible to describe a time scale of ego and identity formation, in which there are, of course, important cultural differences. The first essential consideration is the degree to which the child's constitution is appropriate to the cultural pattern, and the second is that he must experience certain types of situation at a culturally appropriate time in early childhood if an identity is to be formed that is immune from vicissitudes. It is desirable that a child's feeling of identity should become as independent as possible of circumstances.

IV. EMPATHY

Reference has been made above (pp. 6–7) to the emergence of somatic sensitivity and the evolution of empathy in the child through somatic orientation, formation of body image, and body intuition. It appears to us that the problem of empathy is enormously complicated and intricate, and a few examples may be given for illustration and for further discussion. It might be inquired: with whom and with what does the individual empathize? What are the possible relationship extensions of the personality in this direction? What is the relation of empathy to identity? It is not the same as the relationship between empathy and identifying. It has been suggested that this ability to empathize may be one of the most important qualities required of those who are going to work on other cultures. There is a great deal more that needs discussion about the interrelationship of empathy, identity, and identifying. (See also *Identification with Others*, p. 12, and John Donne : 'No man is an island . . .')

Empathy may have other facets, too, such as seeing others as a subject as well as an object. It is pointed out that the organization of identity of an individual may prevent empathy formation, as in caste society in which it would be virtually impossible for a caste-member to empathize with an outcaste. However, this may be broken down by other identities, as in the case of the high-caste doctor; but in this instance the basis of understanding would appear to be the goal of changing the other person.

One man may empathize with another in spite of the fact that the latter is incapable of empathy. So empathy is not necessarily a reciprocal relationship like affective rapport. Empathy can become important for understanding the identity of the other, but there may be a failure in empathy because of projecting into another.

Sex Differences in Empathy Formation

We must consider also an interesting sex difference in empathy formation in the contrasting situations of the female infant who, in normal circumstances of maternal care, grows up to feel like the person who brings her up; and that of the male infant who must grow up to feel different. In the case of the female infant, empathy can develop in relaxation in the maternal relationship, and the resulting development can include not only intuitive empathy, but also intuitive acceptance of differences through the mother's acceptance of differences between herself, the baby, and other babies. In the case of the male infant, this intuitive situation may be largely absent, and empathy will be a later developed or acquired characteristic.

However, while intimate contact with a woman is the standard situation of male infants, whose developed empathy, therefore, will be open, as it were, to differences as well as similarities, many female infants lack intimate contact with a man. Intuitively, they will be open to differences only in so far as they have been receptive to them through the mother. It seems likely that impairment of intuitive empathy formation may particularly involve this element of acceptance of differences, because only in a high degree of empathy is it conceivable that the mother's acceptance of differences can pass to her infant.

It is suggested that this failure, in the case of some girls, of intuitive empathy to include the acceptance of differences, combined with lack of opportunity for its development, may lead to an inability to form a relationship with a man, and thence to a state of inviolable virginity that characterizes the psycho-sexual state of some women. This thought may lead to a concept of impenetrability that may characterize the heterosexual relationship of many women, the effect of which, as a matter of common observation, can be observed in the behaviour of both men and women towards certain women in the social group. The parallel situation in men is rare and may have other psychodynamic origins, e.g. the identification of the man with an 'impenetrable' mother; or identification at an oedipal level.

Empathy and Burial or Cremation Wishes

One curious aspect of empathy can be seen in the wishes expressed by people concerning the disposal of their bodies after death. What is the notion of physical identity that lies behind the gift of the body for research purposes or for medical education? The prevalent notions in a community practising burial in the village cemetery may be markedly disturbed by the introduction of cremation. In the latter there are many variations in the disposal of ashes. Some may wish their ashes to be quickly destroyed, but may or may not want to have a memorial tablet or note in a book of remembrance. Others may wish to have their ashes scattered in some well-loved or particularly significant place, which desire might be one aspect of the search for immortality, perhaps a form of cultural reincarnation? Thus, a man might wish to have his ashes scattered in that place which for him is the most symbolic of his country and so achieve an identity with the culture in death.

In this connection we shall discuss later the kind of people for whom the various aspects of location are important, and the fact that, for some people, death is one aspect of their identity.

V. IDENTIFICATION WITH OTHERS

Identification has been described as one of the earliest and least differentiated steps in the process of identity development (p. 5). Empathy has been defined as the capacity to feel into another (p. 7), and its origin has been traced in somatic sensivity (p. 7), somatic orientation, etc. (See also *Empathy*, pp. 9–10.) There is a link between the amount of empathy possessed by an individual and his conception of his relationship with another person as a whole.

Child-Parent Identification

The child-parent relationship has been extensively studied in relation to identification, and it is obvious that the growing child passes through a number of phases starting with that of the foetus, who presumably has no identity apart from the mother. The infant and toddler are both in a phase of differentiating themselves from the environment, but with increasing maturation of systems of perception and of emotional development a phase of psychological identification with parents will appear. This has been extensively described in psycho-analytic writings. The development of the child in this respect is, of course, a constituent of growth of the family relationship. As growth proceeds, the system of identification will become more and more abstract and will pertain more to the systems of values and way of life of the family and the society than to the parents, and this process will also serve to define more sharply the personality of the individual.

V. Identification with Others

Certain specific situations may influence this developmental process, notably neurotic pressures from parents upon their children delaying and distorting the abstraction of the system of identification. Children of famous people are in a special position in this regard, in that certain elements in their personal relationships and family values may be disproportionately strong and may make more difficult the development of a general and abstract identification along family or community lines. Children so placed may remain in a more infantile state of parental identification, and therefore dependence and imitation; or, alternatively, of negative identification and neurotic independence-seeking.

Friendship, Courtship, and Mating

Friendship, courtship, and mating, normally, are successive phases in maturation of the identification process, and in these phases the tendency towards abstraction will be reversed, to some extent, and the definition of the individual personality may be threatened. In adolescence the individual will commonly seek out a mirror of the self, in forming what might be termed a symmetrical rather than a complementing love relationship. This may help the individual in the definition of his own personality, and this is also true of hero worship, which is a relationship existing in the fantasy of the individual in which a mirror of the idealized self may be formed. Thus the symmetrical friendship of adolescence may help in a common fight for identity when this has been impaired. In this respect, pairing off with the opposite sex at an early age, as will happen in societies in which such is possible during adolescence, may reduce the chances of a mature complementing type of sex relationship.

In marriage there is a potential conflict between the desired identification with the spouse and fear of loss of identity, a conflict which is greatest where the personality is diffused in the sense used by Erikson and where there may be a fear of the dissolution of its borders. To this fear may be added that of loss of identity through the other's image of oneself and the demands of the new relationship. In an attempt to meet the situation, the

Identity

immature personality may strive to maintain the image of the other unchanged, and therefore defined, or else to fit a fixed romantic image on to the love partner. On the other hand, in the relationship among mature marriage partners there is a sustained and continuing process of identification with each other which may be the scientific basis for the notion popular among Philippine Islanders (and possibly held more universally) that in successful marriages the husband and wife get to look alike. The facial similarity has been noted to increase with the years. This phenomenon is equally observed in adoptive children who, in time, may seem just like the composite of their parents.

Over-identification is a trap for the immature in marriage selection, the dangers of which can be illustrated by the case of the marriage of two individuals, both youngest siblings and united in the common fight for identity, who may be faced later with their united rejection of their oldest child. Such people may also be intolerant of change in the partner because it destroys the identification, and may feel that only the past is safe. On the other hand, the search for a complementing relationship may also be a neurotic feature of immature personalities with a sense of inadequacy. This might be considered as a 'mirror' relationship in a distorting mirror. In this case, also, the individual's need for the spouse to remain unchanged may dominate the marriage.

Hatred and Identification

Hatred can be a strong tie between individuals and between groups, and can be illustrated by such concepts as 'my friend the enemy' and formalized in codes of conduct in warfare and in social or professional rivalry. In the last-named case the symmetry of position of two antagonists will complicate their rivalry to the extent that it appears to be possible to have identification at one level of relationship and hatred at another. There are wide cultural differences in the behavioural expressions of these phenomena, for in one society love may be easily associated with anger and in another almost completely dissociated. Of common significance, however, is the attempt to disarm the hatred and feared enemy by identification.

VI. Identity and Group Membership

Extreme Emphasis on Identity Factors

Conversion experiences represent extreme forms of identification with others. 'To lose oneself in order to find oneself' is to become identified with the ultimate in the individual's value system. A Child of God is aware of no barriers with God. (See also p. 46.)

VI. IDENTITY AND GROUP MEMBERSHIP

Group Loyalties

The extent to which the individual feels responsible for what other people are doing gives a clue to his degree of identification with those people. We might first consider the difference between those communities in which everything is related to one central value and those in which this is not true. Speaking in broad terms, one might say that it is part of the Anglo-Saxon way of life that identity tends to be distributed centrifugally, as it were; so that a man will belong to such a district, such a family, and such a religious sect simultaneously and in parallel. The effect can be compared very interestingly with the extremely integrated positions taken up by some small national groups, particularly when they form racial minorities. Thus it could be said that there is a tendency for, for example, Irish, Scots, and Poles living abroad to relate everything to the central value of being a member of their race. This is probably not an inborn characteristic, as far as the race is concerned, but rather an effect of the social dynamic.

Group Prejudice

Strong in-group loyalty feeling is one aspect of prejudice formation against other groups (see also *In-groups and Out-groups*, p. 19) and in this connection and from general principles it is possible to deduce a method of fostering a strong in-group loyalty feeling. This would be by bringing selected influences to bear on children, and this is done in many small minority communities, particularly when the basis of the in-group distinction is religious. We shall take a hypothetical example from a long-dead religious controversy, in order to avoid rousing objections from members of a current religious party. Let us suppose that, at the time when the Manicheans were an active religious community, a mother belonging to that persuasion wished to ensure that her child would grow up a loyal member of the faith, she could not do better than relate all behaviour values to the Manichean position. Thus good actions and good behaviour of which she approved would always be referred to in such terms as 'that's a good little Manichean'; encouragement in times of difficulty and trouble, 'be brave like a little Manichean'; and bad behaviour would be stigmatized, 'that's not worthy of a Manichean', and so on. Then, provided that the basic identification of the child with the parents was positive, an ineradicable prejudice in favour of all things Manichean and against the rest of the world would be built up. One might add that this position is not without its dangers in that, if the basic identification contains negative as well as positive features, there is a possibility that the child will rebel against the system and reject it. (For a discussion of self-hatred in minority groups see also Gordon Allport (1954), *The Nature of Prejudice*.) Such rejection, perhaps, is the biggest single factor in schism formation in religious groups. The negative aspect of such prejudice formation is well illustrated by the case of the drunken father whose son becomes strongly anti-alcoholic; out of the rejection of identification with the father-figure is born a life-long prejudice against the agency that is credited with making his father what he was.

For further study is the subject of the formation of identity in members of special communities, such as religious sects that have either been displaced or have moved by design. The rigidity of social patterns that may evolve is suggestive; as shown, for example, by the Hutterites of certain districts of the middle-west of Canada and the U.S.A. In writing on the scientific study of multiple loyalties, Guetzkow (1951) has outlined research areas in the field of definite relationships between hierarchies of loyalties.

Laughter

It will be relevant to consider here, briefly, in connection with cults and closed value systems, two aspects of laughter – laughter *with* and laughter *at* another person or object. The capacity to laugh *with* appears to depend upon the image of the self in relation to another, i.e. upon capacity for empathy; but, in contrast, laughter *at* something else or another can be a defence mechanism against anxiety and hence of aggressive or hostile significance. This is possibly a classic difference between humour and wit – the former pertaining more to empathy and the latter more to defence or aggression. The relationship between empathy and humour is not simple and direct, because the existence of empathy does not necessarily imply the possession of a sense of humour, but it may be true that laughter *with* is impossible without some degree of empathy, and it is also probably true that when empathy is above a certain pitch of intensity the capacity to laugh *with* will disappear.

The point may be illustrated by the case of the circus clown, or, say, Charlie Chaplin. Most people with a moderate degree of empathy will laugh *with* the clown as he goes from trouble to trouble; they will find him comical, but perhaps at the expense of a feeling of pathos. A minority, lacking empathy, may laugh *at* the clown when the situation provokes an anxiety/defence reaction. Still others, with more intense empathy with the clown, find his difficulties unbearable and anything but a laughing matter.

In human interpersonal relations, people laugh *with* their friends. In group relationships the situation may be comparable, for within a cult or closed value system empathy will be considerable, and laughter between members considerable also. But at moments of more intense empathy, such as solemn religious ceremonies or party crises and the like, laughter would be impossible and is inconceivable. Likewise, members of the closed value system are incapable of laughing *with* non-members in anything even remotely connected with the system. If their empathy is restricted to others within the system, which is not uncommon, they will stand out as being completely humourless, but they may and probably will retain the capacity to laugh at non-members or other systems, in the aggressive/defensive aspects of laughter.

Identity

Roots

A most important aspect of identity consciousness is the question of roots. It seems unlikely, for example, that one can be a world citizen without having a root somewhere. Therefore it will repay the study of the conditions necessary for an individual to be able to grow up, or settle down, in his identity. The question can be asked, 'What relation is there between earlier and later loyalties and in what order do they come?' If this is put in practical terms, the question is: under what conditions does a child expand his system of loyalties from the village to the district and out-wards to the country and the world, or contract them from humanity down to the village?

There are many questions which may be asked about roots, e.g. must there be a place? But this is probably too topographi-cal, for a sense of at-home-ness may be developed that has little to do with topography. Some families will create a constant home environment wherever they are living; in others, the sense of home may be quite disturbed by repeated moving. There are almost infinite numbers of variations possible; e.g. one family that travels extensively may always keep the children with the parents and yet have a home, to which they return from time to time, that serves as a root for the whole family. Another family may be static in one place, and yet send all their children to boarding-schools, but preserve a strong sense of family loyalty and at-home-ness. The different types of behaviour met with among these various families do not suggest, necessarily, that family life is stronger or closer in one or the other, but instead that there may be tremendous variations in strength and quality of home attachment that may be related to the development of different kinds of identity. In one respect, it might be thought that the difference between the two families quoted is an aspect of total family identification in the respective cultural patterns.

Leadership

Of all the facets of identity, perhaps those of individual and social environment and their interrelationship are most important.

VI. Identity and Group Membership

Many subtle factors can be studied in the phenomena of leader and led, including the interrelationships between the led. For example, what is meant by leadership? The first significant point is the identification of the members of the group with the leader, with which is associated the identification of the leader with the group and the interpersonal relationships of the group members. There are many varieties, e.g. among the Nazis, identification occurred with each *Führer* and the hierarchies within the party had very definite personal elements. Russian Communists, on the other hand, have their most important identification with the party and, on the strength of this, they are expected to be able to criticize the leader of the particular echelon.

To take an example in the U.S.: the phenomena behind membership and leadership may be even more complicated than the foregoing, and there may be a hierarchy of identity in the case of small ethnic groups which are under the pressure of the majority towards acculturation. Children in such situations may find it difficult to identify with their parents; and a not rare tendency is for children to turn away from their parents and to form gangs. A child will not uncommonly become the leader of a gang of younger children. Anna Freud, working in England after World War II, has described phenomena encountered among one-time child inmates of Nazi concentration camps, who had lived in a small child community with minimal contact with adults. There was a hostile rejection of adults, and the development of an intensely close community organization and interdependence of a most rigid type (see Freud and Dann 1951, also Soddy, 1955, Vol. I, pp. 146–148).

In-Groups and Out-Groups

The possibility must be considered of in-groups and out-groups, in which different values are set on the relationship of the individual to the group. These concepts have in common the dimension of a social distance, which will often be related to social role. A group in relation to another group may be higher or lower, or mobile, moving upwards or downwards. Such groups have in common negatively toned devaluations of other groups, and in

Identity

this way are quite important instruments in the social paraphernalia. The strength of the reaction of group members to the interpolation of non-members can be regarded as a symptom of the in-group/out-group situation and as a rough measurement of the strength of group feeling involved and of the degree to which the group composition is open or closed.

Reference Groups

In addition to the group of which the individual is a member, other groups can be used to set a goal, provide a standard, or supply an audience, in a positive or negative way. This leads us to the concept of the reference group or groups. A reference group might be defined as a group to which the individual refers his behaviour. This does not exclude the individual's own group from being his reference group. One aspect of the social reference group is 'keeping up with the Joneses', which, though it is one of the important mechanisms of social change, is a negative connotation, in that it derives from the fear of falling behind. The reference may even be the standard of the group to which the individual would like to belong. Reference can also be the method by which the individual in the group identifies with the group as a whole, i.e. identification with the ideal.

Morality

There is a moral element also in the positive or negative evaluation of group relationships, but, whether positive or negative, in some sense all groups of reference are included in the main group, because as soon as any group reference is brought in the 'non-reference' has to be brought in also.

It might be objected that scientists can make a greater contribution if they talk in terms of science and not of morality, but moral decisions cannot be alienated from the property of science, even if no more than related to the decision about and responsibility for what a scientist studies and produces.

It cannot be ignored that identity is closely tied up with concepts of superiority and inferiority, or positive and negative judgments; and these may constitute mental health problems.

VI. Identity and Group Membership

For example, if a boy is defined as *not* a girl, this has a strong negative meaning. It is seen more clearly in the remark, 'I am an American and *not* a foreigner', in which all foreigners are devaluated to some extent. There should be a world of difference between saying positively to a child, 'Behave yourself' and saying, 'Don't behave like a baby' or 'animal'; but in common usage it must be admitted that 'behave yourself' is often used with the concept that the child is behaving badly and should stop behaving badly. This is linked with the point already made about inculcation of prejudice.

Identity Change

Both positive and negative factors are implied in other forms of identity change, such as change of social class, marrying out of social class, change of nationality, and change of name. Identity changes of these kinds often imply both a rejection of a former identity and the positive moving towards another; and in the instances quoted there may be a large element of forming a new positive identity, especially in those cases in which the old identity was rejected by the individual. There are striking cultural differences, of course, in this respect, and as far as the change of name is concerned, the problem is far from simple. For example, when an immigrant to the country has a name that appears outlandish and unpronounceable in his new country, he will commonly modify it so as to be nearer to the new cultural norm. This may be sound social sense and common sense and it may also be evidence of a genuine advance in the process of acculturation and identity formation. But it probably always implies some change in the individual's identity. However, before one seeks closure on this idea, it will be necessary to study what effect change of name has on identity. In the Philippines there is a belief among less culturally advanced groups that changing the Christian name of a sickly child will improve his health. Or again, an author writing under two or more names may say that this has an effect on his whole style formation. There may even be an occupational or artistic mobility in this respect. This effect on style becomes clear in cases of psychodrama where gross deviations are temporarily lost as identity is changed in the dramatic role. (See also *Social Conventions permitting Changes of Identity*, p. 45.)

It is clear that in a society in which women take their husbands' family name upon marriage, there will be marked differences between men and women in respect of name changes. Strong group pressure towards a change of name will affect the issue, and this brings into relief the fact that all these factors under discussion should be considered in the light of the reciprocal or dual nature of identity, i.e. the interrelationship between the individual and the group and social environment in which each individual lives.

As a cultural example can be cited the Chinese reluctance to change the surname. A man would almost never do so, and it is something of an insult or a joke to ask a Chinese to take another name. Even children would seldom be put in such a position, and this is one reason why widows are very reluctant to remarry. Traditionally, adoptive sons are selected from the nephews of the same surname, from the nearest relatives to the more distant ones, so there would be no need to have the surname changed. When a woman marries, she becomes 'Mrs. So-and-So', but when she signs her name, or on her visiting card, she retains her own surname – with or without the addition of the husband's surname above her own, as should be done in accordance with proper modern legal practice. Quite frequently, she is still called or addressed by her own maiden surname and personal name, especially by people who knew her in her own parental family. As a teacher, she is often registered still as 'Miss So-and-So', or an expression literally meaning 'one who is born earlier' may be used for a teacher of either sex. This has come to be a polite form of address for educated persons of either sex.

Individuality and Group

In *The Time Scale of Ego and Identity Formation*, p. 9, we have referred to identity strength and ego strength and have advanced the idea that they can be antithetical in some circumstances. Ego strength has been seen as having some relationship with individuality. At this point we might take up two further aspects of group feeling: the strength of group feeling in relation to the self in isolation; and in respect of relationship with other groups. The former can be assessed through attitude of the group to new members and to death of members, and the latter in terms of positive and negative group attitudes. We have already discussed the role of the reference group in defining identity. In discussing a subject, a man may say, 'speaking as an Englishman . . .' (or as a freemason, or a governmental official, or a farmer) and it may be that antithetical attitudes are implicit in all these possible social roles. Here we are nearing the problem of individuality and group. Further discussion of some ethnological aspects of this subject will be found under *Some Ethnological Considerations,* pp. 34–35.

Individualism and Collectivism

Among the religious convictions of people, what might be termed their elective identifications, there can be seen interesting divergencies of systems; e.g. in Christianity there are two antithetical positions in regard to relationship between the individual and the group: the emphasis on salvation by faith and works; and the antithetical salvation by belonging. The latter represents the collective or group approach to human existence and in such concepts as the 'guilt of creatureliness' – the partaking of all in the sins of humanity – there is the apotheosis of group feeling; the individual in his ideas of guilt is identified with creation.

On the side of individualism there is, in rapidly changing and developing cultures, a strong pressure on the individual to increase individuality, and with it the sense of personal responsibility essential for successful adaptation to changing conditions. The importance of further study of this field cannot be overestimated in the case of previously static cultures that have become subjected to technological change. Much the same can be said of cultures with a fixed system that are subjected to vast population movements and similar upheavals.

At the opposite extreme is the pressure to decrease individuality characteristic of closed value systems, whether they be religious or political. In a religious closed value system there may be great pressure on the individual to live as a saint, and though he will not be created a saint until after his death he will, in fact, have died as a saint. For those who perhaps do not achieve saint-hood, it can be said that, whatever they do in life, they must die within the religious system and there is great pressure and great anxiety that the full rites should be completed before death occurs. Dying outside the reach of religion is to these people the great irredeemable tragedy. Recognition of the existence of a similar motivation makes comprehensible to outsiders the notorious political treason trials of recent years, which have been concluded, after conviction, by confession and recantation. The individual at the last is true to his identity, whatever his devia-tion may have been, by dying in the movement; it may be thought that the person has carried the collective ideal to the extreme by making a human sacrifice of himself.

Naturally, these matters will take on very different forms in societies in which there is a belief in reincarnation, and in which the whole system of living and dying may be very different. In China and among the Chinese in Hong Kong, Christians will generally think like those of the same faith in Western countries, but a large proportion of these do not entirely give up the tradi-tional practice of 'remembering' (commonly erroneously called 'worshipping') their ancestors. This is done both at the graves and at the family shrines or photographs. The graves are usually visited twice a year, at Easter and at Christmas, if they are Christians; if not, then at the 'Ching Ming' Festival in the spring, and at the 'Chung Yeung' Festival in the autumn. An added reason for these visits to the graves is to see that they are in good state of repair. The occasions for remembrance at the family shrine, where there is either a tablet or a photograph of each departed ancestor, are generally the anniversaries of the birth and the death of the ancestor. However, this is discon-tinued after the hundredth anniversary of the birth of the ances-tor concerned. There were probably two main reason for this discontinuance, the first a practical one, because by then those descendants who remembered them from first-hand knowledge would be few, and the more spiritual one for those who had any belief in the reincarnation of the soul, because it was popularly believed that by that time the departed soul would have either gone to Heaven or passed on to some other existence. This is a mixture of 'ancestor worship', Buddhism, and more popular faiths and superstitions, mixed in varying proportions from family to family, and varying from one member of a family to another. Likewise, there will be vast cultural differences, both in the religious and in the political world, according to whether the commitments concerned involve an observance once a year or permeate every part of the life of the individual. An illustration of some of the curious aspects of this subject is the pressure felt by Chinese to have a son, in order that there shall be someone to carry on this act of *remembrance,* which is supposed to enable the soul to be at peace, and so that the family – and the family name – might be perpetuated. If no son is born to them, the matter can be put right by adoption, and it is of interest how different will be the feeling of the individual after he has gained **his son.**

VII. FURTHER ASPECTS OF IDENTIFICATION

How are Individuals Identified?

Returning to the various facets of identity, we shall now consider the relative strengths of drives towards, and to avoid a goal. An illustrative question might be posed: Which is the more important to an individual – the family from which he came, or the family which he formed himself? There are subtle differences in family life raised by the issue, e.g. a mother of six children may, when she refers to 'home', always mean her own childhood home which perhaps broke up twenty years previously, and not where she is now living and bringing up her own children. What effect could this be expected to have on the family atmosphere and on the children's identity formation? Within a culture important differences can be anticipated in this respect also.

Two important interrelated questions arise (a) How do individuals identify themselves? (b) How are they identified by others? Here we would like to offer a number of situations for further consideration. Some people identify strongly with their belongings or their properties and, in doing so, become very vulnerable. To others, location is all-important, and this might include the place of birth, the place of family origin, the place to which the individual feels he belongs now, where he hopes to go, or where he fears he may or may not be going in this life and after death. In addition to the cultural variations, there are many possible situations to be considered: e.g. that of the child whose parents bring it up as an offering to or future member of the parents' own childhood families; that of a child whose parents bring it up as a future member of their own (forward-looking) family; and that of the child whose parents bring it up to become in due course a member of its own independent marital family.

In the traditional Chinese family, the individual was identified more as a member of his family, his clan, and his village and district, and less as an individual with a separate identity. With urbanization and the breaking up of the large family into smaller units, the individual and his immediate family circle has received more attention, and now there are people with varying identities in different circumstances. For instance, when some older member of the clan dies, the obituary notice would often include a mention of all male members of his clan, some of whom would hardly ever be considered in everyday life. Also, when two Chinese met in a distant province or in a foreign country, they would feel a closer affinity if they should have come from the same village or from the same province. Even now, in country districts, it still sometimes happens that a whole village are members of the same clan and therefore have the same surname, the married daughters having gone off to live with the families of their husbands in their own villages. These customs of inheritance through the male line have made the position of the woman very insignificant. A daughter or a wife had no rights of inheritance from the father's or the husband's estate, if he died intestate, though she was entitled to maintenance, and the daughter was also entitled to a dowry if she married.

Death is a further aspect of identity, from the point of view

VII. Further Aspects of Identification

both of the individual's own identification and of his identification by others. Some people reach their main identification by the death they died. But, on the other hand, there is a strong tendency for human beings to wish to die their own death. By this is meant a desire to live out one's life, and not to have any extraneous event cut it short.

Labels

The matter of identification by others also bears on the question of 'labels', which, broadly speaking, refers to the designation of people by others. For example, an individual might become strongly identified with his social label of 'Professor'. He might be able to operate only in a milieu in which his professorship was recognized. In a social situation in which is professorship was not relevant, where his 'label' did not mean anything, he might be quite unable to adjust himself. On the other hand, in the case of another individual, a multiple role might cause no conflict and the professor might move from his role in the university to that of a cummuter, spectator, father, etc., with no difficulty. This again brings the argument round to the fact that identity is a continuum, that its loss is not an all-or-none phenomenon, nor can it be compartmentalized. The 'label' is essentially a function of the environment, a distinction mark that is attached to the object in question. Identification with the 'label' by the individual implies identification with his identity, the point which has been discussed above in raising the question of 'settling down in one's identity' (see *Roots*, p. 18). An example of the unfavourable operation of this would be the causation of delinquent acts by labelling the child delinquent and getting him thereby to expect delinquent acts of himself. The possible multiple labelling of an individual, together with the continuum that his identity represents, leads on to the question of hierarchy of identifications with identity and thus to hierarchy of identities. (See pp. 38–40.)

Some of the subtleties of variation that are possible can be seen in naming practices. For example, in some families there is a limited number of names, from which parents may select, for their children. In other families the custom is established that the oldest son always holds a certain name, or he may be named after his father or grandfather. Elsewhere, a newly born child may be given the name of a dead relative. Conversely, parents may have an urge to give their child a new and entirely original name.

The study of the use of first names in different cultures throws up important differences. There is a story applied to many American situations: a nursery schoolboy in the U.S.A. who was asked the surname of his friend Billy said: 'I don't know him well enough to know his last name.' In contrast, a distinguished foreign visitor to the U.S.A. may set a problem to all his acquaintances, because no one knows when to call him by his first name, and he himself may become bewildered in this process. If he is called by his first name when not ready for it, he may well feel that this is an invasion of privacy, which is resented in many cultures, and not only by people of high status. An example can be quoted of an actual case of an individual having to lose his identity (if that was symbolized by his surname) before he could become a full member of the group. A war-time British temporary staff officer in the Indian Army (at that time partly officered by the British) had to attend a periodic staff conference of which the other members were all regular army officers. For about eighteen months he was the only member who was always referred to by rank and surname. But one day, after the most senior officer present unexpectedly used his first name, he became a member of the group in a way in which he had not been previously.

In traditional practice a Chinese often had several names, which was very confusing to his friends and acquaintances. As a child he might have a 'pet name', sometimes also a 'school name', but there was always a regular, ordinary 'name' which generally consisted of two characters, one being common to all his brothers and the other personal to himself. Some large families would have the same common name for all male members of the same generation in the clan, so that at a glance it would be easy to identify the 'family rank' to which he belonged. No matter what the relative ages might be, a person would always have to refer to as 'uncle' or 'great-uncle' another belonging to the generation of the father or grandfather. Similarly the daughters of a family would all have a 'common name' combined with a personal one, though it was seldom the practice to use the same 'common name' for female cousins. In recent decades some families have given expression to their conception of the equality of the sexes by using the same 'common name' for their daughters as well as their sons. The 'common name' or 'rank name' became a sort of 'classifier'. When a son got married, he was also sometimes given another 'big name', which was carved on a tablet and decorated with red cloth and placed in a place of honour in the household, but he seldom used this name. On the other hand, he would often choose for himself another name which we might call the 'name of address', as his friends and acquaintances are supposed to call him by this one, it being regarded as impolite to call an adult person by his regular name. In traditional Chinese custom it is regarded as disrespectful to use the name of a person more senior than oneself, which is just the opposite of the Western custom of having a child named after a person as a sign of respect to that person, as is now sometimes done.

Identification in Families

A similar cultural and social problem is met within ordinary families when a newly married couple has to find a solution to the problem of what to call the respective parents-in-law. In line with the inferior position given to women in the traditional Chinese family, the daughter-in-law was expected to address her 'in-laws' in the same way as the servants did, whereas the son-in-law was allowed to call his wife's relatives in the same way as she did. This practice also is now dying out, and in modern families husband and wife call each other's relatives in the same way as the spouse does, e.g. 'Father', 'Mother', 'third elder brother', 'fourth younger sister', etc., or by name. It is interesting to note that in China there is a very distinct expression to describe each type of family relationship, and people can at a glance discover exactly how two people are related, once the relationship is mentioned. The expressions 'cousin', 'uncle', 'aunt' are differentiated into the various categories of such relations, e.g. 'third paternal elder uncle' or 'fifth maternal younger aunt', etc., so that the exact person can immediately be identified. The solution to the problem of what to call parents-in-law, when not prescribed by cultural form, is influenced by subtle differences of identity within the two families concerned.

Identity as an Interpersonal Phenomenon

The illustration in the preceding paragraph brings emphasis to the fact that, in many respects, identity is an interpersonal phenomenon. Previously the thought has been expressed that identity is a quality which an individual presents to others; perhaps now this thought might be expressed again in a different way, that among the factors that go to make up identity are the qualities that individuals present to each other. For further discussion we can suggest : identity and its relation to identification with the parent-figure; and the importance to the formation of identity of the group membership of the individual. The latter has already been touched upon above, pp. 19–22.

VIII. FURTHER CULTURAL FACTORS AND IDENTITY

Social Role, Status, and Class

As an exercise, it is important to inquire wherein lies the centre of individual identity, in a particular culture as compared with other cultures. For example, in one culture the generalization might be true that the role, or in particular, the social role, is a major part of the individual's identity. In a second culture, the social status may be the most important aspect, and in a third, perhaps social class.

The distinction between social role, status, and class is a fine one. One definition is that social role is a dynamic aspect of social status, i.e. what people are expected to do in their status. Social class implies a place in the social structure or even a position in a hierarchy. In one country any professor of whatever origin may command respect; but in another country, of two professors the one that comes of a recognizably higher social class may command more respect. This attitude carried to an extreme would result in a comparatively uneducated man of a higher social class commanding more respect than a highly educated professor of low social origin.

It is a common European phenomenon that a whole social class, for example, the working class, shows a remarkable solidarity of aspiration; and a child in such a system will be completely identified with it and at home in it. Social ambition in such a case will probably lead the child, on reaching adult life, to the desire to improve the social status of the whole class. It is probably true that in other countries, in North America and elsewhere, the desire of the individual family to improve material conditions and family status may be much stronger than any concern about class status.

As an aspect of family aspiration, the present state of the family must be related to the concept of future career held by the family members. This may be illustrated by the phenomenon of the high professional ambition that is commonly met with among immigrant minority groups. Comparable phenomena are also important in cases of internal migration, for example amongst university and city business people. In a highly developed culture a 'back-to-the-land' movement is often seen, in which highly sophisticated and town-dwelling people are obsessed with the notion that the only life for the children of the family is life on a farm. The practical issue in any of these types of family is the desirability of a greater awareness on the part of the parents of the child's possible need to choose his future life sphere for himself. Phenomena of family aspiration relate also to the possibility of a hierarchy of identities in the same individual and this point will be taken up more thoroughly below (*Hierarchy of Identities,* pp. 38–40).

Some Peer Culture Phenomena

We shall now consider the existence in many cultures of small cultural subgroups based on age. There is a remarkable cross-cultural similarity in some of these phenomena in different Western industrialized societies, particularly among peer-group cultural phenomena of which zoot-suits, Teddy-boy clothes, and so on, are outward and visible signs. They sometimes become fossilized, as it were, and remain on in adult life in uniforms and modes of dress. An example of the institutionalization of these phenomena can be seen in the rigid social patterns of boarding-schools in an old-established cultural pattern being subjected to rapid technological change, as in the case of nineteenth- and twentieth-century Great Britain. In this example the change is twofold, both amongst the boys and girls who are developing from childhood to adulthood, and in the culture as a whole.

Petting and necking practices originating in North America, but now spreading to many European countries, are characteristic of youth in transition from childhood to adulthood, in a society in which control or leadership by adults has lapsed. It is typical of societies in which petting practices flourish that they themselves are rapidly changing. It appears that in place of identity in the family group, the teenagers in a changing culture develop another identity with the age-group in order to secure personal protection.

At a level less integrated into the culture there are the phenomena variously associated with zoot-suiters, Teddy-boys, etc., referred to above, which appear to be widespread among the youth of modern cultures in transition; and which flourish among that section of teenagers which has emerged from the family shelter and has not yet established itself in the adult world. Groups of adolescents organized in this way and known as *Edelweiss* groups are known to have appeared in Germany following the 1919 disturbances. After World War I a youth movement in Czechoslovakia adopted many of the dress and other customs of American cowboys. The 1930 depression in the U.S.A. gave rise to similar youth activities, culminating in the zoot-suit, and in more recent times adolescents have found expression in jive-clubs and rock 'n' roll. In the U.K. the Teddy-boys dress in a prescribed uniform, caricaturing the fashions of the first decade of the twentieth century (reign of King Edward VII). In Australia they have the name of 'widgies and bodgies', and in the Philippines, 'low-waist gang'.

VIII. Further Cultural Factors and Identity

Closer examination of these groups reveals a number of interesting common features. First, and most important, they represent the sociologically unestablished or deprived and, secondly, the psychologically dispossessed, for these groups attract those who have outgrown their own family ties, but have not yet been assimilated into the adult cultural pattern. Thirdly, they have a very strong urge to establish identity with the peer group and must develop a distinguishing mark, to achieve which they use the simplest of bodily materials, such as dress, haircut, and general physical appearance. Fourthly, essentially this is a pre-heterosexual movement, and the curious fact is that each sex exaggerates the dress characteristic of the other and, in addition, each is primarily concerned with its own sex. These tendencies are quite marked, e.g. both in Europe and North America, boys' dress tends to have narrow shoulders and broad hips and generally shows off the body-line. Haircut takes a more feminine form and there is in general a dandyish preoccupation with clothes, choice of colours, and so on, which is feminine rather than masculine in the present age, though this would not always have been so. The girls wear trousers and sweaters and have a more masculine type of hair-do.

Nationalism

Nationalism is a phenomenon of identity with the nation, to which is also related the phenomenon of 'we' and 'they' groups. However, there are striking cultural differences between various peoples as to how this may work out, e.g. as we have already considered (under *Group Loyalties*, p. 15) with some smaller national groups that have travelled widely and colonized extensively, their members, almost to an individual, will invariably be representatives of their nationality foremost; whereas in other groups, where individuals have not the same urge for a narrowly defined identification, an individual at various times can be less of a representative of his nation than a university man, or a soldier, or any other social role that is appropriate to him.

33

Identity

IX. IDENTITY CONTINUITY, COHERENCE, AND FLEXIBILITY

Some Ethnological Considerations

An individual can be said to remain the same throughout life. But is this true of his identity, or does that change? There are numerous interesting illustrations from historical and cultural studies. For example, in Greek mythology of about 2000 B.C. there was a triad system in which a goddess appeared in triplicate, as it were, as an immature maiden, an adult woman, and a crone. She would have a different name or a different identity even in each phase, constantly passing from one into another, but remaining the same person throughout. Another aspect of this paradoxical heterogeneity of identity was the dualist system of the sacrificial king and the tanist: the king ruled during the waxing year and was killed sacrificially by the tanist, who reigned during the suceeding year, but was killed by the next king, and so on. These two were twin aspects of the same identity, and a similar phenomenon is seen in Chinese Buddhism; there are a number of deities, amongst whom is the 'Kwan Yin', who is regarded as a male Indian deity taking a female form and becoming the 'patron saint' of women and children. Many other religious systems show comparable phenomena, e.g. the Christian Trinity. It was typical of Greek thought that the highest value was placed on the integrity or homogeneity of the person, though there might be three or even more co-existing aspects. In contrast, the Hindu and Buddhist doctrine of transmigration of souls can amount, in principle, to a rejection of self and of the integrity of identity. Nirvana is the Hindu doctrine of abstract union with the God-head, signifying merging in infinity and loss of individuality; this being a privilege reserved for the very few.

In Bali the transmigration goes round and round within the same family and this tends towards a lack of definition of or possibly a disappearance of identity. Thus, in Bali, there is little sense of the individual meaning of death and no mourning except in the case of young babies, in which case the prevailing feeling seems to be one of exasperation at no result for trouble taken. Misfortune during life is held to be due to the necessity of paying debts owing from a previous incarnation. This vague causality is about as far as cause and effect become apparent to the Balinese. Thus a new baby is welcomed within the family, as a reincarnated ancestor; but, owing to a lack of sense of personality and of causality, the new baby is not identified more precisely than as being a member of great-grandfather's generation; he does not represent that great-grandfather and is not actually identified with him. Hence there will be only ceremonial difficulty over the fact that great-grandfather is still alive, for no attempt is made to match new babies with defunct forebears.

In China, traditionally, as referred to on pp. 24–25, a different emphasis is met with. Here, a man must have a son in order that there shall be someone to carry on the act of remembrance after his death. The Chinese are therefore motivated to provide for the continuation of the family name after death.

Personality Integration

We have to consider further important aspects of the integration of identity, viz. its continuity, coherence, and flexibility. Two illustrations will point out the area to which this refers. First, in the practice of pscyho-analysis it seems that a change of identity may sometimes occur during analysis and when this happens the value set upon integrity of identity may be threatened; and it may cause anxiety in the analysand about whether something had been wrong in his previous system of values. The second example refers to the value set upon the integrity (continuity, coherence, and flexibility) of identity, which will relate also to the hierarchy of identities and the degrees of acceptance of identity (see Section X). Marked differences in the capacity to adapt can be noted in travellers. For example, some people, the moment they set foot in a foreign country, merge more or less indistinguishably into that country. Others stand out rigidly unchanged in the different culture. There is a difference in cultural attitude here: for societies will differ widely in their willingness to admit a temporary stranger or an immigrant into various facets of their culture. They may, for example, be more willing to share their public culture with strangers than their family life, or vice versa.

Identity Strength

Underneath this concept of continuity, coherence, and flexibility lies the idea of the existence of a tendency which serves integration, having a general-manager function. This might be defined as identity strength, and it has been mentioned on p. 9, where it was described as a strength in the sense of a force rather than in that of a building, i.e. as a dynamic, not a structure. One might inquire about the kind of identity strength that leads to good mental health, and as a start postulate that it will include permanence, durability and flexibility. Erikson in *Childhood and Society* (1950a) has discussed the idea that in the U.S. it is necessary to be able to tolerate staying in one place all one's life, at the same time as to be prepared to move tomorrow.

Identity strength, therefore, refers to the continuity of the personality, i.e. the relation of the past to the present and to the future. It is non-changing in that who the individual is going to be is a necessary component of who he was. This may not be true in a changing culture and probably there are special features of ego identity under conditions of change. However, identity management will be an aspect of identity strength, and this leads back to our concept of identity continuity, coherence, and flexibility.

Formalized Ways of Accepting Temporary Breaks in Identity

There are widespread ways in which temporary changes of behaviour involving abrogation of responsibility and, to a greater or lesser extent, a break in identity, can be formalized and made acceptable in society. These will show cultural variations, but can be illustrated by considering the significance of certain commonly used phrases. In Britain and the U.S.A. 'I was beside myself (with rage, envy, laughter, etc.) . . .' signifies a temporary loss of control under extraordinary conditions of feeling in which the individual feels absolved of guilt. 'I was not myself' is felt to be a rather more culpable situation where influenza, a headache,

excessive fatigue, or even mild drunkenness may help to excuse
a lapse. At a more serious level of dissociation of responsibility is
the phrase 'outside myself', in which part of the speaker, as it
were, joins in the condemnation; and in this light also should be
regarded phrases like 'my better nature' or 'my baser self'. In the
term 'possession' there is a demoniacal concept of personality
changes. Also, in less culturally advanced groups in the Philippines, being 'bewitched' (under evil influence) signifies relaxation
of normal control and a surrender to the environment, as in cases
of 'rape with consent'. In a less moral connection, the expression
'sent' is popular among the 'Beat Generation' to signify a relaxation of normal control and a surrender to the environment, as in
rock 'n' roll and jive.

Promotion of Identity Strength

What can be done under current conditions about identity
strength? First, we have to work with what is there already. An
important point of departure will be young marriage and in this
connection the essential factor on which to concentrate is the
suitability of aspiration of the family to the circumstances they
are in. Conversely, there may be a chaos of aspiration that may
lead to ego weakness. We have already discussed on p. 31 certain
cultural differences in this respect.

Prevention of Excessive Strain on Identity Formation

An important corollary of the development of identity strength
is the prevention of excessive strain on identity formation, and
this and the promotion of identity strength can be taken together.
There may be four practical issues:

1. How to recognize the kinds of strain placed on the identification processes by modern conditions, in different societies, or in different stages of change.

2. The initial steps in child-rearing necessary to provide the
   kind of strength needed to prevent identity strain. By this
   we mean the development of such a system of affective
   relationships between a child and his human environment

37

that will lead to incorporation of ideals and moral values. When excessive strain is placed upon the processes of identity formation, hostile or affectionless systems can develop that may lead, for example, to delinquency, drug-addiction, and alcoholism.

3. The extent to which strain can be repaired at different times of life. We have referred to the relation of strain to the identity-formation age, but there are also to be considered various other periods such as passage from childhood into adulthood (see pp. 32–33); assumption of responsibilities, as at marriage; and, strikingly, upon retirement. The well-known phenomena of comparative loss of identity following retirement or loss of political position, and of premature death, are social questions of some magnitude.

4. The related practical issue is to consider all the points at which the community can intervene in setting the style of family life. We have referred to the climacteric periods. Special opportunities will occur at these and at different phases of social change, e.g. in the maternity hospital, the child welfare clinic, in school; whenever children leave home or become institutionalized; following upon separation or divorce of parents; after desertion by, prolonged absence or death of parents; in housing schemes and in the development of new towns; community development and planning of industrial developments; following immigration or emigration; and in the introduction of social security programmes and when the retired person first takes a pension.

X. HIERARCHY OF IDENTITIES

Multiple Identities

It has been discussed how an individual may have concurrently a number of identities, both actual and potential and at different levels of relationship. In any position in society there will probably be an expected range of identities for individuals, though this is not necessarily tolerable in all cultures. In fact, the culture will determine the range of identities that are tolerable and anything outside this range will lead to distortions and the formation of less congruent personalities. There may be a conflict of identities, in which case there will be a need to resolve the conflict from what might be termed a deeper identity position; and there may be many surprises in the outcome in that a particular identity may prove to be more important to an individual than either he or other people think.

Hierarchy of Identities

These considerations lead on to the possibility of the existence in individuals of a hierarchy of identities by nationality, race, religion, occupation, sex, and many other factors, not necessarily in that order (see also p. 5). Not only may there be a hierarchy of identities, but there may be a graduated scale of intensity of identification, comparable with the hierarchy of values within an individual's value system. The possible interplay of the various factors can be illustrated by the hypothetical example of a world congress of a religious movement. In addition to their various identities of the kind mentioned above, the delegates have one common factor that separates them – their nationality; and another that brings them together – their religion. For some, however, nationality may be more important than religious denomination and for others the converse will be true; and these variations in intensity of identity may themselves be continually changing. Another example of the different possibilities that may co-exist in one person can be taken from a member of a committee who will have a certain identity as a father, and another as a university professor, in addition to his identity as a committee member. The relationship of these factors will be governed mainly by individual and independent factors, but they may become very important in conflict situations, such as may occur, for example, from a juxtaposition of Eastern and Western cultures within one family circle.

Hierarchies of identity may be orientated in time, and this

Identity

can be seen in the crazes that sweep countries temporarily. For example, the Davy Crockett craze, which was seen a few years ago in many parts of the world, could bring small boys great joy in being identifiable as a respected figure rather than just John Smith's little boy. It is possible also for an individual to undergo a regression in hierarchy formation within his system of identities, as may happen when an individual, who has previously lived a free and independent life, voluntarily enters a disciplined service. In this case a possible conflict in identity can become resolved in terms of a deeper identity position which has never been entirely resolved, presumably the child-parent relationship.

Religious or political conversion is an example of a replacement or rearrangement of the hierarchy. In either case the hierarchy will be altered and the process may include destruction of previous properties and values. Among the practices of what might be termed extreme conversion cults there are many types of initiation ceremony, of which baptism is one example of a rite in which death and rebirth are symbolized.

The wish of the individual as to how he wants to be identified is a factor of his own hierarchy of identities. Obviously this is subject to great variations, of which cultural values are not the least cause. One might conclude this section by remarking further that, when a total loss of identity occurs, the individual loses his unique place in history.

Basic Plot

We shall discuss later the question of permanent change and dissociation of identity, when dealing with more pathological matters, but here refer briefly to change of identity as it illustrates continuity, coherence, and flexibility. Change of identity may be total; or it may affect only facets; and in either case the change may be permanent or transient. It might be said that it is possible to distinguish between those people who can be *known* in any of their roles, and those whom it is necessary to see in many or all of their roles before they can be *known*. We shall refer to this as the existence of a *basic plot* in the person's life and this concept relates to those of identity integrity and breakdown (pp. 35, 48–49).

Style of Identity

Another way of expressing the idea of basic plot is 'style of identity'. Style or basic plot is the continuity of change of identity that occurs as the person's career unfolds. There are great numbers of questions to be asked in this field. For example, to what extent does an individual change significantly on moving from childhood to adolescence and thence to adulthood and family responsibilities; from schoolchild to student and thence to junior employee, from senior employee to head of the department? What happens to systems of identity when, for example, a person moves from a profession into the civil service? What about the experience of women as they move from the status of girl to those of wife, mother, and widow? These are the natural changes in status to be expected in human life. There are also specific phenomena to consider, such as the effect of the change of name and of identification upon style of identity. The case of those who enter a closed order, particularly of a religious character, is of interest here. It is clear from observation that some people can be recognized in any of their roles; they appear to remain always the same people. Clearly also the variations that occur will depend on cultural style as well as on individual style; e.g. it might be true that all the husbands belonging to a certain nationality behave in a recognizably distinctive way towards their families; whereas in another culture there may be no set style. Not only is it sometimes true that husbands of a *certain nationality* behave in a recognizably distinctive way towards their families, but also husbands belonging to certain regional groups *within a culture*; e.g. differences in the attitude and behaviour of husbands towards their wives among regional groups like the Tagalogs, Visayans, Ilocanos (Philippine dialect groups) are well known.

There are many unanswered questions here, e.g. might it be true of those who are recognizable in all their identities that they do not change because they are essentially unchangeable? To answer this question we need information on the maturation patterns in childhood of such persons, particularly in regard to the time adjustments of the child. Did the child pass from the suckling stage to the toddler stage and thence to the nursery group with a smooth maturation pattern? Was puberty precocious or retarded? An irregular maturation may be responsible for absence of style of identity, or basic plot. Possibly a retardation in or resistance to the maturation pattern during development may be paralleled by an incapacity for or resistance to identity change thereafter. Conversely, flexibility of identity may result from easy, smooth, and regular adaptation in childhood. These are speculations upon which cross-cultural studies may give a clue, and some suggestions for ways of testing the hypothesis that changeability is positively associated with smooth, unbroken maturation are given on p. 50. It has been suggested that children in families brought up by young parents show a greater facility for change of identity in different roles than children who have been brought up by grandparents. It may be that children brought up by grandparents are acquainted with age and therefore more resistant to change, but we must not leave out of consideration the possibility that unchangeability may be deeper than this, and may be constitutional.

XI. UNUSUAL FORMS OF IDENTITY

We have already discussed the changing forms that identity may take within the normal pattern of life, but now we need to go farther and consider some of the extreme cases and reactions that are found, the unusual forms and what might be termed the 'pathology' of identity formation. Here we would note the absence of satisfactory forms of classification, and also remark that such phenomena as lapses of memory, loss of memory, identity breakdown, double personality, family romance, and assumption of new identities might constitute differences in quantitative reactions, but they necessarily also involve changes of kind. This brings us back to the problem of the essentially different levels that the states of health and illness represent.

Change of Identity

We can begin to get some light on the unusual forms of identity through considering some of the strange experiences during the war, where a change of identity was forced upon normal children in unusual circumstances. Anna Freud has described a case of a three-year-old Jewish child living in the Netherlands, whose family was concealed in a Dutch house for three years and compelled to undergo a change of identity and name. The mother impressed upon the little girl that she must never answer to her old name. Under pain of the likelihood of her mother being taken from her if she did not comply, the child faithfully followed the instructions for three years. One of her first remarks on reaching the age of six and grasping the significance of the liberation was: 'Can we have our own name back, Mummy?' This episode might be considered as illustrating an extreme form of identity organization, or integrity, i.e. continuity, coherence, and flexibility.

Migration

In population movements, different effects can often be observed on different members of the family. With a drastic change of environment, the adult men may be disorientated, because they have been forced to abandon their old occupation and their old familiar surroundings and their old public positions and they have no basis on which to make an adaptation to the new. The housewife, however, may find that family duties are essentially similar whether in Bohemia or in Wyoming, and may make an easy adaptation to new circumstances, though the family may in fact make remarkably few concessions to the majority culture pattern of their new surroundings.

In cases of new settlement, and it may be true of the U.S.A., too, the whole population has a great deal of experience of moving both in respect of first- and second-generation immigrants and in the amount of internal migration, which is a constant feature of newly settled countries. It seems that such people tend to visualize themselves as being within a framework of an overall pattern of moving, and moving into one place does not present problems necessarily different from those of moving into any other. It seems likely, however, that this facility of accepting

Identity

movement may disappear from the cultural pattern quite quickly when a settled habit develops, especially in remote rural regions. Psychologically this may be linked with the establishment of a high degree of emotional security in the first year of childhood. It is typical of the moving, unsettled population, where mothers have close and everyday intimate control of the child and his movements, that the identifications of the first-year baby are predominantly in the interpersonal relationships they form. Throughout life, to such people, human relationships may remain more important than place. The converse seems true in the case of ancient settled communities where upbringing of infants may have become more institutionalized and less personal and where place identifications form a relatively more important part of the system. This links up also with the thought on pp. 41–42 that ability to respond to change may be positively related to smoothness of maturation. It is interesting to note that in the organization of the Kibbutzim in Israel, the maturation pattern of the children is the reverse of smooth, in that a sudden change in social and emotional environment will occur when they enter. The subsequent social organization is marked by rigidity.

'Family Romance'

The general hierarchy of identity may be subject to distortion by fantasy as in the case of 'family romance' which, in the view of psycho-analysis, is a fantasy of children that they are not the natural children of their parents but have been adopted. One view holds that the strength of the 'family romance' may be inversely related to the degree of temperamental congruence between parents and children and thus will be dependent on bio-chemical factors. It is also directly related to the child's image of the parental attitudes and seems likely to occur strongly in those cases where there is a wide difference between the intellectual standard of the child and that of his parents.

The 'family romance' looms large among the identity problems of adopted children, among whom it is common to meet with the invention of a fictitious identity, including an entirely fictitious history; or alternatively, an avid search for the natural parent.

XII. More Extreme Forms of Identity Formation

XII. MORE EXTREME FORMS OF IDENTITY FORMATION

At this point we are coming to the edge of what we have termed the pathology of identity formation. At the normal end of the scale there is day-dreaming, which might be regarded as one of the great experimental disciplines of young children. In the case of day-dreaming it is true that a difference in quantity may involve a difference in kind. When day-dreaming leads to absorption in the dream and to a failure to distinguish between the dream coming from within and the impulses coming from without, the phenomenon changes its character and becomes potentially pathological. 'Family romance' represents a more nearly pathological form of day-dreaming which may become quite pathological if the child's sense of reality becomes obscured. From this level of pathology it is possible to go on to consider other extreme cases, as illustrated by loss of memory, extreme conversion reactions, and double personality. There is also to be considered the degeneration of the very old, to whom only their early life is real. These are extreme cases which, when studied in greater detail, may throw light on the process of identity disintegration.

Social Conventions Permitting Changes of Identity

Some identity changes that may resemble identity disintegration may be socially approved. *Incognito* of special personages may be used to protect them, to afford them relief from strain, to allow them to escape temporarily from an assumed identity; to give the society also some relief from formality and to establish better communication between people and ruler. *Nom de plume* is an acceptable social convention also, which may be dangerous and irresponsible, as when it enables serious scientists to write alarming fiction under a different name; but it may protect other authors, and sometimes in the case of scientists and artists is justified on the ground that it provides income while leaving the individual free to pursue more serious but unremunerative ends. On p. 21 we referred to legal change of name in order to obscure ethnic origin, and so on, or to permit rehabilitation after scandal or otherwise bury the past. However acceptable any of these conventional devices may be, their potential effect on individual identity should be borne in mind.

In contemporary life in Western society there is an interesting convention usually termed 'off the record'. In this a responsible person wishes a fact to be known but not attributed to him or to the organization concerned. This, like the temporary identity-changing devices already mentioned, may have elements both of protecting the individual and the public and also of evading responsibility. Study of which individuals use this device frequently, and in what circumstances, might throw light on this phenomenon and the individuals concerned.

Specific Sources of Strain

A point of entry to this field would be to consider some of the unusual strains on the family identity system that may be encountered in modern life. For example, artificial insemination presents a curious problem for the whole family in that the husband of the child's mother has to play out a social role in respect of the child. This can sometimes be supported only by the acceptance or insistence by the whole family, including the supposed father, that the child resembles him.

The experience of identity is closely connected with the body image of the person and specially with the facial expression. It is, therefore, most important to study cases in which a human being was suddenly crippled or paralysed, or had his face mutilated – with the possible result of a severe disturbance of identity, such as depersonalization, or double personality. Conversely, difficulties may arise from operation deformities and after cosmetic operations which change the facial expression considerably. The patients are not necessarily happy, but seem strangers to themselves and take time to become acquainted with their new physical shape. It would be important to study this in relation to different sex and age groups. Likewise the assumption of new identities following upon initiation ceremonies, ordinations, consecrations, taking the veil, and so on; and other stranger forms

XII. More Extreme Forms of Identity Formation

of identity change such as the acts of mutilation that may occur in some cultures as, for example, the one-time practice of *suttee* in orthodox Hinduism in which the widow threw herself on the dead husband's funeral pyre, or other practices of burning alive wives or slaves in some primitive cultures, would well repay further study.

Special Position of Some Individuals and Whole Groups

Actors and dancers are in a special position in regard to temporary change of identity. Often they will possess a faculty of being able to look at themselves from the outside, or actually to visualize their own act as if they were spectators. This faculty is common among children whose emtional needs are not fully satisfied. We would like to refer also, briefly, to the special position of certain whole groups, such as movie actors, gypsies, some groups of American Indians, and many others who have a group-identity role to play out in society. Their situation is as old as that of the travelling medieval mountebanks, and it finds some echo, greater or lesser, in the professional role of many recognized disciplines in modern society.

Double Personality

Much has been written in literature and, especially, fiction about the formation of 'double personality'. This, though dramatic when it occurs, is not common in any well-defined form. It might be thought that children show it to an incipient degree in the 'family romance'. What does the double represent? Healy has described the case of a man who, as a boy, committed murder and who referred to his boyhood self always in the third person. Healy suggested that this represents, as it were, a state of non-identification. A temporary and non-recurrent day-dream of double personality can be seen in the case of acting which, as indicated above, deserves much more study. It would repay attention to study the degree to which the whole of life might become an act to the professional actor, and to gauge the effect of this on the total personality of the actor.

47

Disturbances of Identity

It seems probable that a great deal can be learned about identity from the study of its disturbances, disturbances that are such a marked feature of some types of schizophrenia (though, of course, this mental disease is much more than just a disturbance of identity). Something may be learned from the extraordinary results that can be achieved if a way is found to integrate successfully a schizophrenic patient into some kind of group. For example, a schizophrenic can often show a much better integration in role-playing than in expressing the self. Successful integration depends on more than re-establishing the identity, but it is likely that there can be no integration without identity. In practice, the main difficulty is to find a group into which the individual can be integrated, and a means to achieve the necessary identification.

Some disturbances of identity are shown up clearly in the older studies of hysteria. Janet (1920) described a range of hysterical phenomena that might extend from no more than absentmindedness to a condition of multiple personality in which the individual might have several almost complete identities. The question would arise, is this a sign of strength or weakness? And, perhaps, the answer depends upon the capacity of the individual to integrate his personalities, but it will also depend on cultural demands. It will be strength in certain societies. It might possibly be a strength in an individual growing up in a society undergoing rapid change and showing culture lag (see *Continuity, Coherence, and Flexibility*, p. 34).

XIII. IDENTITY BREAKDOWN

Depersonalization

Clinicians are familiar with the concept of depersonalization. This has been described by Martin Roth in the case of children with extreme experience of exposure to contact with death. To what extent does depersonalization link up with the 'body image' and thus with the child's adaptation to the environment?

XIII. Identity Breakdown

The interesting question of mirror identity is relevant; how does the individual relate to the face in the mirror or to photographs, moving pictures, and portraits? The phenomenon of loss of memory has been mentioned above in connection with the formation and integration of identity. It could also be a sign of the threatened breakdown of identity.

De Levita (1961), a collaborator with Rümke, brought to our attention his interpretation of the *Metamorphoses* of Ovid as identity crises. He illustrated this from the story of Phaethon, the son of Apollo, who showed 'family romance' in his fantasies of his origin which, being confirmed by Apollo, resulted in over-identification with his father and an assumption of the latter's role, with Apollo's unwilling consent. But the tragedy was that he was too light.

Attitudes to Death

Death of the individual occasions a crisis in identity rather than a breakdown. In death an individual passes from one phase of identity into another and his state in the latter phase will be much subject to cultural factors. In principle this process of identity passage is hardly different from that of birth. There are three important fields for study here:

(a) the attitude of various people to death;

(b) the concept of dissociation and integration implied in the attitude; and

(c) the identification with aspects of the personality (or the Jungian concept of persona or anima).

Identity breakdown is, of course, closely, if in a way inversely, related to the individual's attitude to identification, and here, too, there may be interesting and subtle cultural variations.

49

Identity

XIV. MENTAL HEALTH IMPLICATIONS

In conclusion it will be useful to recapitulate some of the points
that appear to represent emerging concepts and those with immediate practical mental health interest.[1] The first point that
emerges might be described as the *Principle of Positivism,* as
expressed on pp. 20–21, e.g. that a boy should be brought up
positively to be a boy and not to be something that is not a girl.
This ties up with the question of strong in-group feelings, the
'good little Manicheans' referred to under *Group Prejudice,* p. 16,
and the question of prejudice formation under *Group Loyalties,*
p. 15.

Next we come to the question of identity strength (pp. 36–
37) and the prevention of strain on identity formation (p. 37).
Associated with this are the conditions necessary to enable the
child to grow up and settle down, as it were, in his own identity
(*Roots,* p. 18). Here also there is an important question posed
about the relation between a child's earlier and later loyalties,
which ties up with a speculation on pp. 41–42 that capacity to
change may have a direct relationship with the smoothness and
unbroken nature of the child's development pattern. Rigidity
may come from unchangeability, which in turn may come from
broken development. This important speculation needs testing,
and, among ways of doing so, the following are suggested:

1. Studies of later behaviour of communities in which a major
   part of one generation has been seriously uprooted in childhood by war, occupation, deportation, or emigration, etc.

2. Comparative study of social history of two more or less
   comparable communities in which change occurs (*a*) by
   evolution and (*b*) by revolution.

3. Selective studies of upbringing by grandparents, middle-
   aged and young parents, siblings, and servants.

[1] It has been pointed out that conclusions drawn from the foregoing study
of identity do not invalidate the normal legal procedures adopted in many
countries to establish the 'identity' of individuals, though they may cast
doubt upon the validity of many legal principles concerning responsibility,
and the like.

XIV. Mental Health Implications

Related also is the important question of the relationship between identity and identification with the parent-figure (*Identity as an Interpersonal Phenomenon*, p. 30), and in the same paragraph, the importance of the group membership of the individual. From this we can move to consider further a possible relationship between the persistence of static cultural patterns and collectivism on the one hand, and the association of changing cultural pattern and technological change with individualism on the other hand (p. 21). A very practical family mental health point is the need to consider the child's need to exercise choice (p. 31).

Less related points, but requiring further study, are: leadership (pp. 18–19); the effect of change of name (p. 21); the question of 'family romance' and its relation to adoption (p. 44); the phenomenon of acting (p. 40); the effect of initiations, ordinations, etc. (p. 46); and the further study of more pathological phenomena on a wide range, such as cultural mutilation ceremonies (p. 46); or the reintegration of schizophrenic patients into groups (p. 48); and many other comparable phenomena.

REFERENCES

ALLPORT, G. W. (1954). *The nature of prejudice.* Cambridge, Mass.: Addison-Wesley.

DE LEVITA (1961). Voor de identiteitsproblematick. *Ned. T. Geneesk.* **1**, 96–103.

ERIKSON, ERIK (1950). Growth and crises of the healthy personality. Symposium on the healthy personality. Supplement II to the transactions of the fourth conference on *Problems of infancy and childhood.* Ed. M. J. E. Senn, New York, Josiah Macy, Jr. Foundation.

ERIKSON, ERIK (1956). The problem of ego identity. *J. Amer. Psychoanal. Ass.* **4**, No. 1, Jan, 56–121.

ERIKSON, ERIK (1950a). *Childhood and Society.* New York: Norton.

FREUD, ANNA, & DANN, SOPHIE (1951). Experiment in group up-bringing. *Psycho-analytic study of the child*, Vol. VI, pp. 127–168. For another paper on this material, see *Mental health and infant development.* Ed. SODDY, K. (1955), Routledge and Kegan Paul. Vol. I. Special experiences of young children particularly in times of social disturbances (pp. 141–160).

GUETZKOW, H. (Ed.) (1951). *Groups, leadership and men: research in human relations.* Pittsburgh, P.A.: Carnegie Press.

HARTLEY, E. L. (1946). *Problems in prejudice.* New York: King's Crown Press.

JANET, P. (1920). *The major symptoms of hysteria.* New York: Macmillan.

References

KLUCKHOHN, C., & MURRAY, H. A. (1949). *Personality in nature, society and culture.* Chap. 2. Personality formation: the determinants (p. 35). London: Jonathan Cape.

MEAD, G. H. (1934). *Mind, self and society.* Chicago: University of Chicago Press.

MURPHY, GARDNER (1947). *Personality, a biosocial approach to origins and structure.* New York: Harper.

RIESMAN, DAVID (1952). *Faces in the crowd: individual studies in character and politics.* New Haven: Yale University Press.

SARBIN, T. R. (1954). Role theory. In Gardner Lindzey (Ed.), *Handbook of social psychology.* Cambridge, Mass.: Addison-Wesley.

SODDY, K. (Ed.) (1955). *Mental health and infant development.* London: Routledge and Kegan Paul.

Mental Health and Value Systems

AN INQUIRY INTO THE COMPATIBILITY OF
CONTEMPORARY MENTAL HEALTH CONCEPTS
WITH VARIOUS RELIGIONS AND IDEOLOGIES

EDITORIAL NOTE

THOSE paragraphs in the text which have been indented include material contributed by members of the Scientific Committee of the World Federation for Mental Health, individuals attending conferences held during the course of the project, and other colleagues and friends. In these paragraphs we have also included the committee's discussion of matters of speculation and other matters where full agreement was not possible.

The Scientific Committee does not hold itself responsible for any statement which appears in an indented paragraph. We consider that this material is of interest to the student of the subject, whether because of the nature of the contribution made or because of the individual who made it. In some cases the discussion shows that the committee disagreed with statements which, nevertheless, are considered to be of sufficient interest to the reader for inclusion.

For those paragraphs which are not indented the committee is happy to assume a collective responsibility. Although each one of us will probably disagree at least with some of the statements that are made, we are unanimous in presenting these discussions for the attention of the student of this important subject.

Introduction

AT THE beginning of Study No. 1 on 'Idenity', it was stated that the Scientific Committee of the World Federation for Mental Health intended to publish a series of introductory studies, from an international and interdisciplinary point of view, of basic concepts used in the field of mental health. It was further stated that there were three possible objectives in mind:

1. To seek clarification and, if possible, consensus in an internation and interprofessional sense on the more frequently used concepts in the field of mental health;

2. To review those concepts which appear to be emerging and gaining in importance;

3. To draw attention to those areas patently requiring further study.

It has appeared to many people working in the field, that mental health is increasingly becoming a value, in a similar sense to the modern concept of bodily health. If this be truly an emerging concept, then it is time to consider the relationship between mental health and the established value systems of people.

BACKGROUND TO THIS STUDY

Study No. 2 is based on a series of discussions and small conferences that were held during the years 1957, 1958, and 1959. Interest in the topic has arisen out of the widening scope of international work in the field of mental health and of the problems which occur when the experience of work in one part of the world is transported across cultural boundaries and applied to other types of society.

Mental Health and Value Systems

Mental health workers often encounter resistances and unexpected failures, and some unexpected successes too, when they apply ideas taken from other parts of the world. Up to the present there has been little attempt to organize the knowledge about those concepts and practices in the field of mental health which have a more general validity and those which are strictly limited in location and time.

Since religions and ideologies in various parts of the world differ widely both in essentials and in practice, it may be inferred that concepts of right and wrong, of good and bad behaviour, of virtues and vices, and of ideals may differ also in their content. It may also be inferred that the concepts of mental health and of mentally healthy behaviour among different peoples may differ likewise. This study is an attempt to investigate some of the ways in which concepts of mental health will differ or agree according to prevailing religions or ideologies.

We considered two possible approaches to this subject. The first would have been to call together people skilled in and representative of the great religions and ideologies for an exchange of information about the concepts of mental health which they hold. This procedure, we thought, would be unsatisfying from the point of view of those who are professionally interested in mental health, because of the lack in general of scientific knowledge about mental health among religious scholars. The alternative was to call together from a number of cultures people who, though mainly experts in mental health, were drawn from some of the great religions and ideologies.

The second approach, although more practicable, has certain disadvantages. We could not expect to find people who were equally expert both in the human sciences and in religion. We have consulted mainly with people who are well trained in one or more of the mental health professional disciplines, and who were brought up within one of the great religious systems. This has resulted in an uneven representation of the various religions, partly because individuals from Buddhist, Confucian, Hindu, and Islamic countries were not only less available to us for consultation, but also have been generally less exposed to modern

60

concepts of psychological medicine and mental health. Those that are available have usually been trained in Western centres of teaching, which may tend to make them less representative. A further disadvantage has been the presence of a majority at all our meetings of people who have either come from Western Christian countries or else have been educated and have lived and worked mainly in Christian societies. The majority have therefore been very familiar with Judao-Christian ways of thought and values and, on the whole, have not been specially concerned to discuss their common attitudes, but rather to learn more about those of others. This situation has resulted in many aspects of the Christian position being taken for granted rather than being stated explicitly. It would have required an impracticable lengthening of this work, both in preparation and in writing, to have attempted to redress this balance.

The practical difficulties of our undertaking, therefore, have been very considerable. The first approach appeared to us to be impossible and we have adopted the second, while freely conceding its many disadvantages and shortcomings.

It will be seen, therefore, that this study is primarily about mental health and the ways in which the concepts of mental health that are acceptable to people brought up within the various great religious and ideological systems agree or differ. Our concern has been not with religion, as such, but rather with the views of religious people about mental health. This is not an essay on comparative religion.

Our work method has had to be determined by the availability of personnel and by the limitations inherent in any plan which depends upon getting people together, from various parts of the world, for a series of meetings. The main task has been undertaken by the members of the Scientific Committee whose names are set out on page vi. It will be seen that all the members of this committee belong to the so-called 'Western' cultural pattern. In addition, we have at various times consulted individuals who have greater knowledge of other religions and ideologies than is represented on the Scientific Committee. Thanks to the generosity of the Hazen Foundation of New Haven, it was possible to hold two conferences, each composed of about twenty people, in New York, and in London, respectively, at which a great deal of background work for this study was done. At these conferences viewpoints were presented from within Buddhism, Christianity, Confucianism, Hinduism, Islam, and Judaism. We have also had the help of an expert on Russian Marxism, and of a psychiatrist from a culture where primitive animistic cults exist alongside Christianity and Islam. The final stages of editing were greatly assisted by a grant from the Council of International Organizations of Medical Sciences which enabled the Scientific Committee to meet.

It appeared to us that a systematic representation of defined religious positions would be impracticable. In Christianity, alone, there are many distinguishable trends, each of which would need due presentation. The same applies to all the great religions; it could not be held that an Islamic representative from Egypt could speak for Pakistan, for example, any more than a Christian from Denmark could speak for Peru. There is the additional difficulty in the method that we have adopted, that it may be very misleading to compare the statements of, for example, a Christian of a particular denomination about Christianity, with the statements of a non-Russian, non-Communist expert about Russian Marxism. These and many other difficulties we have noted in the hope that they may be resolved eventually in future studies.

We have taken only the broadest of religious categories for discussion, and of the many political ideologies in the world today we have selected only one for mention. As will be seen below, our main criteria of what constitutes a 'great' religion or ideology have been: first, provision for a wide range of human potentiality; secondly, passage from one generation to another; and, thirdly, ability to cross the frontiers of culture. It might be asked, for example, why a recently popular cult like Existentialism has not been considered? This is because it has shown no evidence, so far, that it is viable, that it will not disappear like many other such cults as its protagonists get older.

This document, therefore, consists of a report on a series of discussions, edited and processed further by the Scientific Committee of the Federation. In it we have sought to open up the subject and to display some of its many facets for further practical exploration. We are asking questions rather than attempting to answer them. We are very conscious that we have not included an adequate list of references and a bibliography. The literature in this field is now quite voluminous, though much of it consists of opinion and discussion rather than fact. Not to have produced a bibiography of sources is, perhaps, regrettable, but to attempt this would be a major task in itself and far beyond our resources.

Members of the committee have attempted to bring to the discussion their knowledge of the literature and we are grateful, too, to those who have attended our discussion meetings for sharing their experience with us. In a few places we have made a specific reference to activities within the Federation and, occasionally, in amplification of points made by members of the committee. On the whole, views and opinions are quoted anonymously, for the committee took the further position that it is better to examine ideas critically than to attempt to present a catalogue of what other people think.

The reader's attention is drawn to the prefatory notice that the views and opinions which have been quoted and to which, in some cases, we have added a comment have been set out in indented paragraphs. Many of the views set out in the indented paragraphs were contributed by members of the Scientific Committee and also by those who so very kindly gave of their time and effort in coming to our various meetings. We thank all those who have helped us in this way and we appreciate greatly what they have done for us. They will know that we agreed not to refer to their views by name; otherwise the discussion might have been stifled by excessive caution, since many of their contributions would be easily identifiable. Though we have withheld their names, we warmly acknowledge our indebtedness to our friends who have helped us. It is certain that the committee, by its own unaided efforts, could not have developed a discussion of a range at all comparable with what follows.

Mental Health and Value Systems

THE SELECTION OF THE SUBJECT

We have referred above to the spread of mental health work across cultural boundaries. At the same time, in many countries, the emphases in mental health work have been shifting away from programmes of therapy and social amelioration towards studies of how to strengthen interpersonal relationships of people, so as to promote a greater capacity for adaptation and emotional growth.

It appears to some of us that the modern concept of 'mental health' is now in an emergent institutional form with a fluid conceptual structure and wide variety of practice; and we are concerned with the question : how far is it exportable?

The prevailing religion or ideology of a community may be regarded in many senses as both an expression and a source of its value system; and it is an important consideration, as the exportation of mental health concepts becomes common practice, to consider what mental health concepts are relevant to people of different religions and ideologies. We therefore decided to examine the compatibility of some contemporary mental health concepts with various religions and ideologies.

A second consideration is that, in much of the mental health work which has crossed cultural frontiers so far, it has been the apparent aim to bring to the people concerned a standard acceptable in the culture in which the workers themselves have been trained. When change and development are widespread, it may also happen that the concepts of mental health that are being exported to another culture will already have become outdated in their culture of origin.

THE GENERAL AIM

It seems to us to be inadequate to attempt to bring people to a point at which the members of another culture have already arrived. Instead, we would advance another general aim, in principle, that mental health concepts should be exported in a

64

way that will get people moving so that they can then set their own direction towards goals of their own conception.

Together with the acceptance of mental health concepts, we must also consider the resistances. Here an interesting comparison can be made with the acceptance of the notion of physical health. The latter has not always been regarded as a 'good object' but, although the operative description of physical health may be scarcely less vague than that of mental health, in recent years and in many parts of the world, physical health has become increasingly recognized as important and valuable. In some countries the notion of mental health provokes such resistance that it is either not understood, or even conceived in terms of its opposite, as public attitudes often demonstrate.

If the concept of physical health as a 'good object' has been acceptable only with difficulty, that of mental health is likely to provoke even greater resistances. Indeed, the concept is comparatively new to most people and it cannot yet be expected that all people will find it 'good'. Such attitudes of non-acceptance, wherever they occur, constitute problems which mental health workers must study when introducing mental health principles.

CROSS-CULTURAL APPLICATION

As the few examples given on pp. 70–72 of attempts to define mental health show, culturally-bound thinking greatly obscures the cross-cultural application of mental health concepts. It is central to our purposes to discuss how much cultural loading, as it were, can be transported across cultural frontiers. One approach is to compare the concepts of mental health, whatever the terms in use, that are characteristic of certain religions and ideologies with one another, and to identify the common ground and also the important differences. Another approach is to take the most widely held ideas of mental health in Western European and North American cultures and identify what aspects are not applicable in certain selected cultures. For example: in a modern industrialized and rapidly changing society there is a great value set on the ability of each individual to be independent and to adapt freely to changing circumstances. Anyone in such a society who shows marked dependence and rigidity might conceivably have the state of his mental health called in question. But in a slowly moving rural community with a relatively unchanging way of life, aggressive independence and the need to experience change might likewise be questioned.

Our discussion needs to take note of the size and extent of the community, culture, religion, or ideology to which the individual has to adapt. Are only those who are capable of living harmoniously in a nation-wide collectivity to be regarded as mentally healthy? What is the position of members of a small minority group or members of a small religious cult? For example, the Dukhobors and the Hutterites and many other small groups have had ways of life that have been regarded by the larger or host community in each case as eccentric or even psychopathological. What is the mental health status of the individual belonging to one of these special minority communities which accepts a certain style of behaviour, but living in a society which rejects it?

THE RANGE OF THE PROBLEMS

The range of the problems that we are studying can be illustrated by a few generalizations made about the major religions. These generalizations, which have an overall usefulness rather than a specific validity, show the extent of the possibilities of variation in what is considered to be mentally healthy. For example, among the great Eastern religions there is a general tendency to teach that the individual should accept external circumstances as they are. The control of the environment by the individual is not regarded as of the highest value. There is, perhaps, more concern with the harmonization of the individual's own inner life and, *pari passu*, with adaptation to the external environment. In Buddhism, human desire is regarded as something to be not only controlled but eliminated. In Buddhist ethical values there is great emphasis laid on taking a 'right view' of circumstances. Taoism goes even further than Buddhism in a direction of non-attachment. Taoism emphasizes withdrawal from competition, the negation of personal effort, and the glorification of 'non-being'.

The emphasis in Confucianism falls more on collective organization and the maintenance of prescribed systems of family and other social relationships. On the other hand, Hinduism has carried fixed forms of social organization very far, but among those who are within the caste system fluidity is achieved by a belief in reincarnation. Definite judgments on actions are hard to form when an individual is thought to be under the influence of past lives and likely to be a different character in the next life, and when there is also a belief that the individual cannot escape his fate. Whereas consistency may be a very important value in a Christian society, for example; in a society in which there is a belief in reincarnation the notion of consistency may not apply. It might be asked, with which of his lives and characters is an individual to be consistent?

The Hebrew religion, with its emphasis upon the conquest or control of circumstances, is in contrast with the prevailing spirit of the great religions of the Far East. The concept of the universal omnipotence of God and of the relationship of God with a chosen people would appear to be reflected in relationships within Jewish families which have a considerable affective strength.

Christianity, like Judaism, has laid emphasis on the affective strength of interpersonal ties and on loyalty to the group. There are many trends within Christianity, and among them will be some in which a greater emphasis is laid on the relationship between the individual and God, and in others on the relationship of the individual to his fellow men. The point for our consideration here is that behaviour and attitudes which may be regarded as mentally healthy in the former might be regarded as unhealthy in the latter. For example, it might be asked : would the value set by society on unquestioning obedience, in a father-oriented society, be the same as that in a sibling-oriented society?

Islam, similarly, teaches that life is a progression through this world towards a more complete understanding of the nature of God – towards illumination. In Islam also there has been a centuries' old conflict between parternalism and the authority of the Prophet on the one hand, and fraternalism symbolized by the Prophet's sons and their competing adherents, on the other.

We have considered a 'great religion' as being a system which provides for a wide range of human potentialities, as capable of being passed on through more than one generation and of crossing cultural lines. It must now be conceded that nineteenth- and twentieth-century Marxism, as developed in Russia, has fulfilled these criteria. Russian Communism developed in, and eventually overcame violently, the imperialistic society of orthodox Russia. The Russians, like other fraternal societies established by violent revolution, have shown a shift of emphasis away from the old paternal authority by enhancing the position of an abstract concept of the collective. Communists, like the members of some Eastern cultures in which an abstraction of the collective is also important, emphasize the necessity of 'right thinking'.

THE MEASUREMENT OF MENTAL HEALTH

In addition to a qualitative assessment of mental health the question may be raised as to how far it is possible to effect a quantitative measurement. At first sight this may appear to be an obscure suggestion which, however, might be clarified by an analogy taken from the study of nutrition.

Nutrition is a state that can be assessed qualitatively, but the success of any attempt at quantification will be dependent upon the amount of available scientific knowledge of the principles that determine a state of good nutrition. What is more, the principles of these basic sciences are, on the whole, exportable across cultural boundaries, and can be applied to the securing of good nutrition just as much in one part of the world as in another, however much food habits may vary.

Therefore, the application of knowledge derived from the appropriate basic sciences can be used to raise standards of nutrition, and to this extent it may be deemed feasible to quantify or measure nutrition. The point for our inquiry here is whether, in the field of mental health, the application of knowledge derived from the appropriate basic sciences might not be used to raise the level of mental health. In this way the notion of measurement or quantification can be introduced legitimately.

Returning to our analogy, it is generally accepted in the public health field that good nutrition is something to work for, but that a state of good nutrition is not an end goal in itself. Most people would consider that there was little value in having a good state of nutrition if the individual was not going to do anything else. In other words, good nutrition may be a sub-goal, but nevertheless it can be important if it is a condition of the realization of higher values than that of nutrition.

This analogy may be applied to mental health which, equally, may be regarded by people as something desirable in itself, but pointless unless the individual is going to do something with his mental health. It is, however, an important sub-goal and a condition of the realization of higher values. We would suggest that good mental health is an instrumental value as well as being valuable in itself, and if this be so it follows that the components of good mental health are instrumental values as well. Just as the components of good nutrition may be measurable according to scientific principles, our problem is whether the components of good mental health are also measurable. There might be, for example, specific forms of education or child up-bringing which lead to attitudes that are mentally healthy in a given culture.

Raising the level of mental health is instrumental in the development of the ideal personality, and it may be possible to implement a cultural ideal by the use of specific scientific knowledge. It is important to keep a clear distinction between levels of aspiration, as exemplified by the concept of 'good mental health', which are instrumental values, and final values which in a given culture might be represented by the cultural ideal as, for example, a saint, sage or hero.

Our next step is to consider more closely the nature of mental health and some of the many assumptions and implications of this subject.

CHAPTER 1

Mental Health Assumptions and Implications

THE NATURE OF MENTAL HEALTH

IT IS customary to attempt to define a subject before embarking upon its study, but the whole of the present discussion might be regarded as an attempt at definition and to do so in brief at the outset will beg the question. We shall begin by giving two assumptions which need to be made explicit – that there can be different degrees of mental health; and that mental health is associated with principles dependent upon the prevailing religion or ideology of the community concerned. Therefore any attempt to define mental health involves consideration of the religious and ideological setting. It is the object of the present study to throw some light on the relationships between concepts of mental health and the notions of religion and ideology.

Next, let us review briefly some of the more recent statements about mental health.

The Constitution of the World Health Organization, formulated in 1947, includes the following:

> 'Health is a state of complete physical, mental and social well-being, and not merely the absence of disease or infirmity ... '
>
> 'Healthy development of the child is of basic importance, the ability to live harmoniously in a changing total environment is essential to such development.'

This definition approached the subject of mental health obliquely by stating that mental well-being is one of the essential components of health as a whole, and that for healthy development capacities for harmonious adaptation are required.

In 1948 the International Preparatory Commission of the International Congress on Mental Health, considering mental health more specifically, proposed a definition that included:

'1. Mental health is a condition which permits the optimal development, physical, intellectual and emotional, of the individual, so far as this is compatible with that of other individuals.

'2. A good society is one that allows this development to its members while at the same time ensuring its own development and being tolerant towards other societies.'

This definition is important in that it brings into consideration the relationship of the individual and society, but it may be thought that the concept of tolerance towards other societies needs further elucidation, because of the complexity of the issues involved.

The question of the role of society in promoting, or even permitting, the mental health of the individual is relevant to the question whether there are states of society that are related to mental health. Two points might be advanced for consideration later: first, for the mental health of its members, a society must provide for perpetuation as well as for growth and development. Secondly, that society is most conducive to the mental health of its individuals which emphasizes the mental well-being of the individual rather than of society; and takes into account the widest range of growth and development, well-being, and safety not only of its own members but also of all human beings.

Returning to the description of individual mental health, it will be noticed that importance is currently ascribed to the essential physical, mental and social one-ness of health and to the concept of harmonious development in a changing environment.

Other people have approached the definition of mental health in a more dynamic way, introducing the concept of the realization of human potentialities; and Rümke (1954) has added the dimension of the value system. Mental health, according to Rümke, includes the discovery of the possibilities and forms which can bring to realization the tendency existing in every man to have a value system that transcends the individual.

In an extended description of individual mental health, Soddy (1950) suggested, among other points, that the healthy mind can meet with ease all normal environmental situations and that the healthy minded person has the capacity to live harmoniously in a changing environment.

'A healthy person's response to life is without strain; his ambitions are within the scope of practical realization; he has a shrewd appreciation of his own strength and weaknesses; he can be helpful, but can also accept aid. He is resilient in failure and level-headed in success. He is capable of friendship and of aggressiveness when necessary. His pattern of behaviour has consistency so that he is "true to himself", and no one about him will feel that he makes excessive demands on his surroundings; his private beliefs and personal values are a source of strength to him.'

The author of the above has discussed with the Committee his present view that this ten-year-old description will be valued only in cultures in which such qualities as adaptation, friendship, legitimate aggressiveness, consistency, and so on, are valued. Rümke has added that it is more applicable to the individual at maturity than during a period of growth.

Interest has now shifted to considering not so much the qualities which go to make up mental health, as how to foster the development of such qualities in people. For such a purpose it is necessary to study which of these qualities and what else besides is valued by people as an ingredient of mental health. When change is taking place, it is not limited to environments or to individuals' behaviour but will also extend to their ideas and beliefs; and it is very relevant to the consideration of mental health to study how the concept of mental health differs in different environments, including those that are changing and those that are relatively static.

We might go on to outline some questions on the nature of mental health, in both positive and negative terms. For example, can a distinction be drawn between mental health and contentment or happiness? Is mental health the same as moral well-being? Is mental health compatible with error and wrongdoing?

Confusion arises from thinking that mental health may equal happiness, and conversely. If this were to be accepted as a formulation, then the term 'mental health' should be abandoned. We take the view that mental health, contentment, and happiness are not identical; and, further, that mental health is not related to single social factors, and is not the same as 'ideals'; on the other hand it makes possible the fulfilment of an aspiration and also can help to secure adequate solutions of emotional conflicts. On the question of moral well-being we might take a position similar to that taken over happiness, i.e. that mental health might make possible the attainment of moral well-being which may in turn reflect upon the quality of mental health. The question of error and wrong-doing we would prefer to leave for later consideration.

The Concept of the 'Whole Man' – Maturity

We have learnt that there is an Islamic principle that health is virtue and virtue is health. The word 'virtue' is derived from Latin 'virtus', which had to do with the whole man, or in other words, the psychosomatic unity of the individual. Thus the notion of human nature is a key concept in identification of what mental health means; and three ways are commonly suggested of conceptualizing human nature: the physical, the psychological, and the spiritual level.[1]

[1] O'Doherty (*Religion and Mental Health*): 'Mental health means a great deal more than mere absence of mental illness. It implies a degree of maturity of mind and emotional development proportional to an individual's chronological age and related to his social and economic background. Mental health calls for integration of the personality, and it signifies judgment freed from distortions due to emotional pressure and, secondly, consciousness freed from obsession with self. Among other things it demands good interpersonal relations with oneself, with others and with God.' See also: definition of health in the WHO Constitution, p. 70 above; and Soddy, p. 72 above.

Mental Health and Value Systems

Levels of Mental Health

The notion of human nature is complex and it is not adequate to attempt to make a simple division between mental good health and mental ill-health; and this is the basis of our first assumption, viz, that there can be various possible levels of mental health. Not only may each level have various components, but also in respect of the different components, the same individual may have reached different levels. An individual might be classified as being of a certain order or level of mental health, but there may be fluctuations over time.

A Hierarchy of Values

There is also the possibility that the individual has a personal hierarchy of values in which mental health represents a value on a graduated range, but related to the range of values of society as a whole.

Objective Reality and Rationalization

It is often stated that mental health includes a sense of objective reality. Here many questions arise as to the nature of objective reality and its relationship with maturity, reality-testing, and so on. On the one hand, it was suggested to us that to accept only the physical world as constituting reality is a repression of the concept of deepest reality; but in another view, the concept of reality does not include subjective mental experience, but only so-called 'objective reality'.

It was also stated that the notion of objective reality can play the role of an alibi, and that sometimes the task of the mental health worker is to help the individual to cease to depend upon alibis that he has constructed. (It was suggested that the mechanism of rationalization is itself invoked as the typical rationalization of sophisticated Western society; we accuse others of rationalization in order to justify our own position.)

Relationship between Society and Mental Health

Many people consider that it is artificial to apply the concept of mental health to society. Instead we would advance for consideration the concept of society being conducive to the mental health of its members to a greater or lesser degree; or, conversely, to their mental ill-health. In the present state of knowledge it is perhaps easier to see evidence of the latter than the former; and regression, deterioration, and disintegration of individual behaviour, and breakdown of interpersonal relationships are among the phenomena cited in this connection.

The prevalence of regressive behaviour might be useful as one index of mental ill-health in society if a scale of maturation were worked out and calibrated, as it were. Any such scale would need to take account of the level of maturation regarded as normal in the society and of the relation between ideals and expectations, both of which would be complicated to evaluate. Adaptation is less useful as a criterion because, as we shall be discussing later, it is possible for an individual to adapt to his own and society's pathological processes as well as to normal and healthy developments. In the case of children, the concept of 'maturity at age' (see Winnicott, 1957) is useful, provided this concept can be elaborated to enable some differentiation to be made between the various possible patterns of growth that are possible in society.

It might be postulated that a society with institutions conducive to mental health is one which has a capacity to integrate the largest number of its members and the largest number of innate human capabilities, and to allow them optimal development. But variations in the levels at which societies function in these regards must be recognized. Different societies may accept lower or higher levels of integration, or permit different degrees of regression or of autonomy, and so on. It is clear that these can never be simple criteria.

(Social phenomena tend to become identified in the mind of the observer with their underlying ideology. This consideration has determined our selection of the value system for study rather than the culture as a whole.)

Social Adaptation and Normality

That mental health and social adaptation are not identical can

75

be illustrated by the fact that few people would regard a person who had become better adjusted as a result of leaving home and moving into a different society as having thereby become mentally healthy. Or take, for example, the case of a small group of 'professional' thieves living in a larger community, and consider the mental health implications to the individual of adjustment to the morals of the small criminal group.

In the past, and still today in some societies, adaptation to society has tended to be highly valued in many societies as a sign of mental health; and failure to adapt has been even more strongly regarded as a sign of mental ill-health. This point is well illustrated by the hypothetical case of an individual who wears no clothes in a society in which clothes are normally worn. He will almost undoubtedly be thought of by the others as mentally ill; but the same individual in a nudist group might not be so regarded by the others. However, different social attitudes do not alter the essential nature of the individual's condition, and it should be remembered that a person's motivation for being nude in a nudist colony might be pathological; and because behaviour receives social approval it does not mean that it is not psychopathological.

There are occasions and situations in which, from the point of view of mental health, rebellion or non-conformity may be far more important than social adaptation. It is clear that no single act should be taken out of context and no single criterion of behaviour used in judgment of mental health. It is the whole meaning of behaviour in the social situation over a period of time that should be considered.

Mental Health and the 'Good Man'

The view was expressed in our discussion that mental health is not an ultimate end, but rather a means to an end which can be valuable or valueless. The possession of mental health is sometimes more or less equated with the optimal functioning of all the factors of the personality, but if a person were to aim at this in order to enslave mankind, this achievement of 'mental health' would not be valuable; it would be evil by the use which he made of it.

Is mental health the same as being good? Some people hold that a man can be very wicked and still be mentally healthy. Take the example of a financial operator in a Stock Exchange or Money Market who had no scruples about making money through the ruin of other people. It is the view of many people that such behaviour is not inconsistent with sanity and mental health. On the other hand, although outwardly the stockbroker may show no signs of mental illness, he is not fulfilling his ordinary human duty if he tries to deprive other human beings, and to that extent he may be considered to have a distorted personality.

If it is agreed that it is possible for an individual to be mentally healthy within any of the great religions, it will follow that the mentally healthy man is not the same as the 'good' man; the content of what constitutes 'goodness' will vary. On the other hand, is it possible to be mentally healthy and be a member of a small exclusive cult? The complications of this question can be seen in the case of small cults that have very rigid standards of 'good' behaviour applicable only to their own members, but which may appear to the surrounding or host culture as amounting to immorality and which frequently exclude the rest of humanity.

The relation between goodness and mental health might be explored, in the direction of the actual capacity of the individual to live up to the ideals of his religion; taking some examples from the various major religions and studying the extent to which the individual lives up to precepts or principles; the community attitude towards failure to do so; and the nature of the conflict aroused in the mind of the individual by failure. Various concepts of the 'good man' can be illustrated by some quotations from religious writings.

First, from Buddhist sources :

'To avoid all bad, to do good and to purify the mind, this is the Buddhist message.'　　　　　DHAMMAPADA

'There are, O Brethren, three roots of demerit, namely, greed, hatred and delusion, and there are three roots of merit, namely, absence of greed, absence of hatred and absence of delusion.'

ANGUTTARA NIKĀYA

'I do not see, O Brethren, any other even one thing, the same as mind, which, if untamed, uncontrolled, brings great harm, and if tamed, controlled, brings great benefit.'

ANGUTTARA NIKĀYA

'Develop, O Rahula (The Four Divine States of Mind, namely), (1) Loving Kindness, by which ill-will will be overcome; (2) Compassion, by which violence will be overcome; (3) Sympathetic Joy, by which jealousy will be overcome; (4) Equanimity, by which wrath will be overcome.'

MAJJHIMA NIKĀYA

'With an axe in his mouth is a man born, with that axe he chops himself, when he speaks badly.'

SAMYUTTA NIKĀYA

From the Sayings of Confucius, we have :

'The subduing of oneself and the return to the practice of the rites constitute Manhood-at-its best.'

'Look at nothing which is contrary to the rites; listen to nothing contrary to them; speak nothing contrary thereto; do nothing contrary thereto.'

'When away from home act as respectfully as you would toward an important guest; handle the people as respectfully as you would the grand sacrifice. Do not do to others what you would not desire yourself. Then you will have no enemy either in the state or in your own home.'

'There are nine things of which Great Man must be mindful: to see when he looks, to hear when he listens, to have a facial expression of gentleness, to have an attitude of humility, to be loyal in speech, to be respectful in service, to inquire when in doubt, to think of the difficulties when angry, to think of justice when he sees an advantage.'

LUN YU, Chapter 15

The Hindu quotation comes from the Bhagavadgita :

'What is the mark of a God-realized soul? . . . How does a man of stable mind speak, how does he sit, how walk ?
When he thoroughly abandons all cravings of the mind, and is satisfied in the self through (the joy of) the self, then he is called stable of mind.
The sage, whose mind remains unperturbed in sorrows, whose thirst for pleasure has altogether disappeared, and who is free from passion, fear and anger, is called stable of mind.
He who gives up all desires, and moves free from attachment, egoism and thirst for enjoyment, attains peace.
Such is the state of the God-realized soul; having reached this state, he overcomes delusion. And established in this state, even at the last moment, he attains Brahmic Bliss.'

Jewish concepts of the 'Good Man' can be illustrated from biblical sources:

'And thou shalt love the Lord thy God with all thine heart, and with all thy soul, and with all thy might.'

DEUTERONOMY VI, 15

'Love ye therefore the stranger.'   DEUTERONOMY X, 19

'Happy are they that keep justice; that do righteousness at all times.'

PSALMS CVI, 3

and from Rabbinic teachings:

> 'Whatever is hateful unto thee, do it not unto thy fellow. This is the whole law; the rest is but commentary.'
> 'Separate not thyself from the Community.'
> 'Judge not thy neighbour until thou art come unto his place.'
> 'The righteous are masters of their passions . . . (they) promise little and do much.'

From Christian precept:

> 'Blessed are the poor in spirit; for theirs is the kingdom of heaven.
> Blessed are thy that mourn; for they shall be comforted.
> Blessed are the meek; for they shall inherit the earth.'
>
> MATTHEW V, 3-5

> 'And though I bestow all my goods to feed the poor, and though I give my body to be burned, and have not love, it profiteth me nothing.'   CORINTHIANS XIII, 3

> 'Finally, brethren, whatsoever things are true, whatsoever things are honest, whatsoever things are just, whatsoever things are pure, whatsoever things are lovely, whatsoever things are of good report; if there be any virtue, and if there be any praise, think on these things.'
>
> PHILIPPIANS IV, 8

From Islam:

> 'Nay, but whosoever surrendereth his purpose to Allah while doing good, his reward is with his Lord; and there shall no fear come upon them neither shall they grieve.'
>
> SURAH-II/112

> 'Lo! those who believe and those who are Jews, and Sabaens, and Christians – Whosoever believeth in Allah

and the Last Day and doeth right – there shall no fear come upon them neither shall they grieve.'

SURAH-V/69

'It is not righteousness that ye turn your faces to the East and the West; but righteousness is he who believeth in Allah and the Last Day and the angels and the Scripture and the Prophets; and giveth his wealth, for love of Him, to kinsfold and to orphans and the needy and the wayfarer and to those who ask, and to set slaves free; and observeth proper worship and payeth the poor-due. And those who keep their treaty when they make one, and the patient in tribulation and adversity and time of stress. Such are they who are sincere. Such are the God-fearing.'

SURAH-II/177

A Hindu View of the 'Good Man'

An Indian Brahmin psychiatrist who was trained in the West, reflecting upon what Hindus regard as mentally healthy behaviour, said that those Hindus who are intensely religious will customarily pray at the temple for help and hope that something will be done for them. He thought that they show few outward signs of neurosis, at least from the somatic point of view. The Hindu who has renounced the things of the flesh and who is then buried alive, having received, as he believes, the word of God, might be looked upon by the majority of his people as divinely inspired. On the other hand, the fact that one man spends his time praying to God does not mean that the soldier who does not is regarded as immoral. In Hinduism there are other qualifications of 'goodness', such as self-control, absence of greed, and not trying to destroy other people.

The above quoted views (which doubtless are not acceptable to all Hindus) of the Indian psychiatrist seem to the Committee to be an example of the near equating of mental health with the

Mental Health and Value Systems

'good man'. There may be a greater measure of agreement with the definition of a great religion as a system that enables men to be 'good'; but we would suggest that it is possible for a man to achieve 'goodness' at the cost of such strain that he might with justification be regarded as mentally unhealthy. Equally we would suggest that it is possible for a man to be mentally healthy within the system of a great religion without being recognized by his community as 'good'. Perhaps it is also true that different kinds of 'good' men can be either mentally healthy or unhealthy.

Mental Health and the 'Bad Man'

Alternatively there is the case of the 'bad' man to consider; bad in the particular sense of one who is not living according to, or is going against, his own system of values. Can such a bad man be mentally healthy? It will probably be conceded that he *can* be mentally ill, and in the minds of many people this will exculpate him from bearing moral responsibility for his badness. But the fact that he may not be held responsible does not make him any the less unhealthy.

While it is unlikely that agreement could be reached on the proposition that all 'bad' people are mentally unhealthy, it might be possible to agree that no 'bad' person could be said to have the highest possible level of mental health, and that many 'bad' people are mentally unhealthy.

Mental Health and Individual Adaptation to Environmental Change

Quality of mental health has no more than a limited relationship to capacity to adapt to environmental change. In the first place, since an individual is exposed to environmental change only in a society in which change is taking place, the capacity to adapt to change can have little or no relevance to mental health in a relatively unchanging society. Secondly, it may be one of the consequences of change in a society that an individual can aspire to a higher level of mental health, which aspiration itself involves changing. In this case the individual's capacity to change will be more relevant to mental health in a society in which such goals of change are consciously perceived and are recognized by the people as being obtainable.

The above should be distinguished from the case of an ideal which is perceived as not obtainable. For example, some of those who advocate mental health work have been known to have an unclear aspiration that everyone should have optimal mental health, and that all mental ill-health should be abolished. Such aspirations in the mental health field are more of the nature of ideals which must always to some degree be unobtainable.

Another aspect of mental health in relation to the capacity to change is that it would appear that in a changing society people who do not change are in more danger of being' in mental ill-health than people who have the capacity to change. The converse situation must be examined also; in a society which does not know anything about change, people who have no capacity to change will not be specially vulnerable to mental ill-health for this reason. On the other hand, in such a static society, although the first people to show change may not be mentally ill, they may be vulnerable to an unfavourable reaction from society. It might be said that the social reformer in a static society is in a dangerous position because of the stress with which he is likely to be surrounded.

Social Adaptation and 'The Good'

It is possible that in some societies social adaptation may be given a more positive value.

A Western-trained Chinese psychiatrist remarked that in a Confucian context it is held that Good is not revealed, or in other words, is not the Word of God. He added that the Confucian ethical system is of a utilitarian kind, and good is social adaptation; there is no organized religion in the sense of the Western Church. Identification with the religion is mainly a matter of indoctrination. Thus, if a child is bad, he is deemed not to have learnt his doctrine well. In a stable society in which Confucian teachings are generally applied, those who adhere to them will be better adapted than anyone who does not. Anyone going against them will be exposed to conflict and the risk of instability may be increased.

One converse of this attitude is that mental ill-health is associated with error and also with wrong-doing. If Good is regarded as social adaptation, then to some extent not to be good is to be in error, because of non-acceptance of the teaching of the institution which has the duty to pass on the moral doctrine.

It is a logical extension of the above quoted Confucian attitude that, in a stable society, to do good is to live in harmony with others, the rest of one's fellow men, for to be in conflict may lead to mental ill-health. In fact the Confucian view, we are informed, is more explicit even than this: good is a matter of social adaptation, and in a sense, Confucian teaching is a summary of the rules of life which make for harmonious co-operation between different members of society. On the other hand, we have discussed the view that merely being adjusted to a society is not necessarily mental health (see pp. 75–76). A person might be adjusted to his society and accepted therein but still, by other criteria, he might be mentally ill.

Mental Health and Social Conformity

The concept of mental health as an aspiration paves the way to a discussion whether it is possible for an individual to have mental health in what might be termed a non-viable value system; that is, a cult or a small minority group, which does not provide for a wide range of human potentiality and which does not transmit from one generation to another. There have been many instances in history of extreme religious cults which have flourished for a generation and then died out. Recently the cult of Existentialism appears to be following this course.

In addition, history has provided dramatic examples of political ideologies that attained great influence, suddenly, and collapsed with even greater suddenness. In recent European history in both the Nazi and the Fascist regimes, attempts were made to promote the mental health of people by exacting conformity to certain ways of life, e.g. the Nazi 'Strength through Joy' movement. It would be consistent with the character of Nazi government, for instance, to adopt a policy with the explicit aim of making all Service personnel as mentally healthy as possible and to prescribe whatever measures that appeared to them to be useful. A less hypothetical example is that of attempts made by the Nazis to 'purify' the race by control of breeding.

Our concern here is with the quality of the mental health that might be promoted by such measures. Aspirations for the human personality realized by the imposition of social conformity will not be valued by most of those who are concerned with mental health in the sense of our discussion.

There is another consequence of social conformity to be considered, in the situation of the Nazi storm-trooper under orders, who had to do much that previously had been strongly disapproved both by society and by the individual. Yet the evidence is that the storm-trooper's actions were approved of by a large number of his generation and socioeconomic level.

We might ask many questions: for example, if an individual storm-trooper were contented with his role and felt secure that what he was doing was approved by his generation, but if he were engaging in practices which previously and within his memory had been disapproved, was he mentally healthy? If not, what other criteria of mental health are important beyond personal contentment, adaptation to current society, and the approval of others of the same generation?

It has been claimed that by no means all storm-troopers were really content; that many suffered from severe mental conflict. War-time psychiatric experience has demonstrated that conflict between duty and self-preservation is a potent cause of neurosis, and also that conflict between different orders of aspirational value will tend to cause breakdown. On the other hand, we understand that many of those who were

storm-troopers before 1939 got satisfaction for their instinctual drives for the first time in their lives.

It is more important, however, for our purposes, to consider
this question apart from issues of war and national survival. We
would suggest that the supposedly contented storm-trooper might
have been regarded as mentally healthy if he had been a member
of a society that had known no higher value system which
included such values as human brotherhood or adherence to
divine law. In those circumstances there seems no reason why he
would not consider himself mentally healthy and also be mentally healthy in the estimation of others in the same situation.

In striving after social conformity, the discrepancy between a
group ideal and the individual's ability to attain it may be so
great as to produce strain that is incompatible with mental
health. Another cause of strain affects people who live in societies
which stimulate certain desires but do not permit their satisfaction or, possibly worse, promote certain long-term aspirations
and do not allow their attainment. An individual's adjustment to
such a society might be maintained only at some cost to his
contentment or satisfaction, because of the strain, conflict, or
tension engendered by his efforts to maintain his adjustment. It
would be legitimate to question whether he was mentally healthy.

If the storm-trooper whom we have taken as an example was
really satisfied and content it could signify that he had relin-
quished certain higher aspirations in order to seize upon a more
limited set of values. We would suggest that if mental health
involves an ability to encompass values, for genuine mental
health an individual's values must not be too restricted as compared with the whole spectrum of which he is aware. When a
whole group of people chooses a lesser value even though it has
at one time known higher values, then the question of mental
ill-health enters the field of discussion. In addition, the matter
must also be considered in the light of the concept of evil.

Social Harmony

The question was asked: if, in a stable society, say, in traditional Asia, an individual were to become consciously Western in attitude, deciding deliberately to change his mode of behaviour so that he was no longer living in harmony with his environment, would he be regarded in his own community as being mentally ill?

It appears to us to be possible, though not certain, that a man's decision to change his mode of life so that he no longer lives in harmony with his own society might in itself be a starting-point of mental illness, but that the mere fact of no longer living in harmony with the environment is indifferent to mental health. It is even possible that a person not in harmony might in the long run change society to his point of view and in the end become in harmony again. Though to be mentally ill may be to be in conflict with one's environment, it does not follow that to be in conflict with one's environment is to be mentally ill.

The important question from our point of view here is, how such a person would be judged by other members of his Asian community. Do *they* think that the individual is mentally ill?

Mental Health and Belief in God

Can any relationship be established between belief in God and mental health, and of the latter with morality and goodness? Religious people sometimes assert that agnostics are less likely to be moral in their behaviour than believers, but this contention is often opposed by people who regard themselves as agnostics. There appears to be no *a priori* reason why an agnostic should not have a high code of natural ethics and live conscientiously by it, but there might be consequences in other forms of behaviour which are not covered by the code of natural ethics. On the other hand, there have also been examples in religious societies of forms of behaviour that are not covered by the code of religious ethics. Some individuals who have no belief in the supernatural are doubtless admirable from the point of view of the moralist; but societies so formed have in the past sometimes accepted practices which are immoral to people who believe in God. It is true also that societies formed of people with a belief in God

Mental Health and Value Systems

have sometimes accepted practices condemned as immoral not only by other societies where there is a belief in God or by a later generation of the same society, but also by agnostic or atheistic groups.

The relationship between mental health, ill-health, and belief in God is far from clear; there is no scientific evidence that in the Soviet Union, which is self-defined as an atheistic society, there is a higher incidence of mental illness or either a better quality of mental health. It would not be surprising to find a higher incidence of neurosis among religious people than among irreligious people, but this would not imply necessarily that their religion had produced neurosis. Possibly their neurosis led them into dependence upon religion.

Social Conformity in Differing Conditions

Every great religion includes a wide variation of cultural pattern together with differing social institutions, and which make also for wide variations in attitude. Islam, for example, like other great religions, spans a broad range of human behaviour. We might ask the question: what happens if a decision has to be made between living the complete ideal human life as put forward by the different Islamic schools, and living according to the principles of mental health?

It was reported to us by an experienced psychiatrist in an Islamic culture in Africa that while an observer from outside might see this situation as a conflict, a person identified with the culture would be more likely to see no particular difficulty in it. It might be that the so-called principles of mental health would not be formulated in the culture as distinct from religion itself. It would be true to say that only general principles are to be found in the Koran, and nothing will be found there about more specific principles of health or of specific items of valued behaviour which have accumulated, in the case of Islam, in the course of fourteen centuries.

Thoughtful and enlightened Moslems do not regard the Koran as an encyclopaedia or a book of divination. We are informed that to them, the scriptures are in essence books of inspiration which, by laying the broad bases of justice and of human relations in general, provoke and stimulate the community to creative action in the light of the spirit of the Book.

It would perhaps be better to take an example from practices which have evolved in cultures that are in process of change, and which, though they may or may not have fundamental religious significance, have acquired a degree of religious sanction.

Let us consider the practice of female circumcision which, we understand, has been widespread in certain African cultures. Most people outside the Arab world will feel that female circumcision cannot be other than a traumatic experience for the girl. On the other hand, it has been reported to us that, in one culture where the practice has persisted, until recently the women have talked about it with pride, a circumcised girl having a different value from an uncircumcised one. However, female circumcision has now become widely regarded through the world as an irrationally cruel practice, and is ascribed to such motives as the domination of women by men. We are told that these critical attitudes are not confined to non-Arab countries but are now spreading among the people who have practised it, with the result that some women are coming to regard female circumcision as a practice imposed by men and, we are informed, many women now feel it to be a traumatic psychological experience. Though their grandmothers and mothers, it is claimed, took pride in having undergone the operation, it is now more and more being recognized to have traumatic psychological effects.

The outsider might wonder whether it is objectively true that it is only recently that female circumcision has begun to be experienced as traumatic by the initiates. It is possible that a more inquiring attitude in recent times has brought the trauma to light, and it might be wondered what would have been the results of an analysis of some of these grandmothers; whether, had comparative studies been made of groups with and without the experience, a disproportionate amount of fear might have been found among the former. It is reasonable to suppose that attitudes change as more and more people become consciously aware of the significance of the procedure and impart their changing attitudes to the subjects of the operation; a process which, however, does not obviate the possibility that the experience has always had some inherent ill effects. The case of female circumcision raises complicated issues not only of social conformity but also of sexual taboo, and cultural history may be a decisive influence. There has been a tendency for outside observers to arrive at facile conclusions concerning the mentality of all those who were involved in the practice without duly considering the complications.

As a possible corrective to the making of facile judgments, we would like to draw a comparison, no doubt superficial in many respects but with some relevance, with the practice of routine tonsillectomy among children.

Let us consider the question, how will a future generation regard the recently widespread practice in many Western countries of removing children's tonsils and adenoids as a preventive, rather than because these organs were incurably diseased? It is being increasingly recognized today that the operation is a mutilation and not without danger, and that the child's experience of being in hospital may have attendant disadvantages. Now that tonsillectomy is no longer considered a routine procedure, parents are displaying more anxiety and concern about the operation, and both parents and doctors are becoming more aware of the children's anxiety. Making due allowances for the communication of parental anxiety to the children, it would still not be a justified assumption that the operation has not always been traumatic, in the sense of inducing avoidable anxiety among children, even if their fears went largely unrecognized by parents, or unexpressed by children.

The centre of this question is, what happens to the effects of such extreme social conformity when conditions are changing in society? In regard to female circumcision, what has changed nowadays is that along with the increasing recognition of the rights of women the imputations of sadism that are made about the practice are being communicated increasingly to the people concerned. In the case of tonsillectomy, the previous generation of surgeons rejected the suggestion that this operation might have lasting traumatic psychological effects. However, nowadays more methodical investigations of children have confirmed what has for some time been apparent from experience of analytical treatment of adults, viz, that tonsillectomy can have a deep traumatic effect on developing attitudes, including those of sexual life.

It seems that the situation in regard to these practices is not essentially different from those other controversial social practices, capital punishment and corporal punishment. Indeed, there are many elements of similarity. It has been the experience in many countries that corporal punishment has been accepted by society and even regarded as a 'good' until such time as cultural changes have taken place. Then as more and more people have become aware of attitudes and customs existing in other countries, of other ways of behaving than their own, some have become liberated from the strict ties of unquestioned social custom. Then, in an atmosphere of greater capacity for social evolution, among other things the rights of children may become increasingly recognized, at which time imputations of sadism and cruelty may be made about such practices.

The disturbances of mental health that arise when old practices fall into disrepute come mainly from conflict of aspirations. The old practice will persist in a relatively unchanging society and could be evaluated there as more or less conducive to mental health in a non-aspirational sense; but when mental health itself becomes a more defined aspiration that may be in conflict with social conformity, a great change in attitude may occur towards practices hitherto acceptable.

Socially Unacceptable Behaviour and Suffering

The fact that in many countries people can be sent to mental hospitals through action initiated by the police and confirmed by the judiciary may indicate that in these places mental illness is sometimes closely associated in the public mind with antisocial behaviour, though the converse of this is not often true. It is common experience that mental abnormality will result in socially unacceptable behaviour, that is, behaviour which the ordinary citizen will not tolerate. The link between mental ill-health and disapproved behaviour cannot be denied but this is not to say that they are synonymous. In many instances the attitude of society will be that the disapproved behaviour is a contravention of positive law rather than unethical or immoral.

Socially unacceptable behaviour is likely to bring unhappiness or even suffering in its train for all parties concerned, and it is a question of some importance to consider the attitudes of ordinary people to the abolition of unnecessary suffering.

> In the course of our preliminary discussions the point was made that wrong attitudes to others may be the source of unnecessary sorrow, and though it is neither possible nor desirable to abolish the tragedy of life, it is a duty to diminish all unnecessary unhappiness.

What is implied by the 'tragedy of life' will be discussed further below (pp. 159–60). Here we shall take note of a different point of view, which is often held, that suffering can also be a perfecting process. Some peoples hold that suffering is an essential part of human life; that it is the means, properly used, to bring about better human beings, if the suffering be accepted.

The operative word in the above indented paragraph is 'unnecessary', and different religions vary widely in their attitude towards suffering.

This is a controversial subject, but it is likely that general agreement could be obtained to the proposition that mental health is not synonymous with the absence of suffering.

Social Attitudes to Wrong Behaviour

Rational behaviour defined operationally is behaviour that can be recognized as not distorted by emotional pressures. It is not to be confused with the rational justification of behaviour, or with the finding of a conscious explanation, in psychology more usually termed rationalization.

All religions deal with the concept of evil and are, to some extent, concerned with differentiating between right and wrong. There appears to be a considerable possibility of divergence between a 'religious' and a 'mental health' point of view in relation to wrong behaviour that seems to be rationally determined. We would like to examine this proposition further, starting with behaviour which is considered by religious people to be wrong but which is also thought of as cold-blooded. If it were established that the decision to do the wrong deed was made coldly, clear-headedly, and logically, it is probable that all religious people would regard the action as evil and the perpetrator as morally culpable. Some might wonder also whether the action did not indicate a defect in mental health.

An instructive example to discuss is the controversy which we are informed has been going on in Great Britain about the cunning, calculating criminal who has chosen a life of crime deliberately, and who is often stated in the Courts not to be mentally ill. The legal question is, to what extent should the man be held responsible in law for his behaviour? The legal and moral attitudes are usually clearly defined – so long as the man is not regarded as mentally ill he must be held responsible. The psychiatric attitude will often differ from this. The psychiatrist may be interested in the very fact that the man concerned has made a cold-blooded choice of a certain course of behaviour which is defined as wrong. This, to the psychiatrist, might on occasion be evidence of a psychopathological attitude, perhaps arising from impoverished interpersonal relationships. The psychiatrist might argue that, when an issue is considered too coldly, divorced from its emotional relationships, the very coldness of the decision might be evidence of serious mental ill-health.

The type of behaviour to which we have referred as cold-blooded is, of course, not synonymous with rational behaviour. Moreover, it appears to us that the concept of judgment not distorted by emotional pressure[1] is not a simple unity; it includes at least four modalities: First, sometimes behaviour that is apparently rational is genuinely so, e.g. when rational choice has been exerted in full response to and in control of the emotions. Second, other behaviour is clearly irrational, as when judgment is distorted by direct emotional pressure. Third, some behaviour that is apparently rational is, in fact, the result of emotional pressure that is distorted because of a complex that inhibits part of the individual's full affective response to the situation. In this case, the individual's judgment may have a quality of coolness that resembles rationality, because it may lack those normal affective components that have been inhibited; in other words, the behaviour has been distorted by indirect emotional pressure. The fourth possibility is that rational behaviour may result from a relative weakness of affectivity, as in the case of the psychopathic personality devoid of affection for others. It is this last type of behaviour that is most likely to be thought of as 'cold-blooded' and its distorted character most easily recognized, in spite of apparent rationality, at first sight.

Culpability

It is likely that all religions are concerned with individual responsibility for actions and culpability, and these questions will also become psychiatric problems in countries where psychiatrists are required to advise Courts of Law about legal responsibility.

Among Christians we believe it to be generally accepted that a person who is mentally ill is less culpable, to the extent that his mental illness is handicapping him, than a person

[1] See p. 73, footnote.

who is not mentally ill. Serious problems of assessment of degree of responsibility constantly arise in cases where the demonstrable handicap is only partial.

The question as it concerns the individual is not simple, but it becomes still more difficult when a whole community or sub-culture is involved.

In the discussion, the case of the Nazi storm-trooper was again raised. It would appear that, as far as the leaders were concerned at least, the Nazis deliberately chose to do what they did; and having been exposed to other values individually during childhood, it might appear to the outsider that they were the more culpable for this reason. However, it appears that many Nazis did not regard themselves as having rejected their early moral training and as having accepted a lower level of morality. These appear to have felt that they were inspired by a new and noble idea of what a man should be. Many thought that the level of morality and ethics in their unit was the highest that they had ever known, and this they experienced as high morale.

Most psychiatrists would regard the behaviour of the Nazis referred to above as not mentally healthy. From a moral point of view, most people, today, would say that it was evil. However, it is legitimate to regard the behaviour as both unhealthy and evil.

Returning to the more general question of culpability, the Roman Catholic view would be that a man can be to some extent emotionally distorted and have his judgment impaired and passions determining his behaviour; but if he knows that what he is doing is wrong and consents to doing it, he still has a responsibility for it. If he is psychotic however, he is not held responsible for what he is doing. The individual is held responsible for acts only to the extent to which he can judge reasonably about them.

As we have discussed on pp. 93–94, the psychiatric view is that in disturbances of mental health reason may suffer as much as, or even more than, the emotions. Though a man may still retain some reason, this does not remove the possibility that he is mentally ill.

We should like to inquire to what extent the statement is true cross-culturally that if a man is to be condemned for an act he must have been aware that there was a rational decision-making aspect to it. One possibility for divergent views arises from the fact that in some cultures and ideologies the individual is held responsible for what he does, whereas in others society as a whole, or a particular sub-group, is held responsible. Therefore, there will be many possible different ways of evaluating the personal, rational decision-making process, according to whether it is so defined in a given society that the individual is held to be responsible, or whether society, the environment, fate, or any other agency should be held responsible.

Repudiation of Wrong and Relationship with Parent Figure

There is a process, which may be universal, in which human beings, after consideration, will repudiate some aspects of their behaviour. It is not known whether there is any culture where that process does not occur, although the sanctions and the form of the repudiation vary.

Among the possible forms of repudiation can be distinguished rational judgment, rational judgment supported by a feeling of guilt, and feelings of shame, sin, or hurt pride. These different sanctions have been associated with different cultures, on the one hand, and with stages of development, on the other.

With regard to stages of development, Erik Erikson (1950; see also Riesman *et al.*, 1950; Mead, 1950; Gorer, 1959) has put forward the notion of an earliest stage of basic trust versus doubt, which is associated with a feeling of sin and includes the possibility, in extreme instances, of the development of a feeling of absolute worthlessness. A second stage, in which the child's problem is autonomy, is characterized by the sanctions of shame – fear of appearing in a negative light to others; and pride – hope of appearing in a positive light to others. Associated with the next stage – 4–6 years – is a sense of guilt, or failure to live up to the standards of loved and/or feared parental figures which have been incorporated into the child's consciousness.

It is probably true that every great religion has a characteristic position in regard to sense of wrong-doing.

For example, from a Christian theological point of view, shame has some relationship to the Old Testament concept of theocratic guilt.[1] Christian theologians have also developed the concept of mature or justified guilt, which finds an echo in psychiatric thinking.[2]

These few examples give some indication of the complexity of attitudes to be found in human concern with wrong. The most striking aspect of concepts of shame and guilt is the universal nature of awareness of transgression.

Toleration in Society of Deviant Behaviour

In the sense used here, the term 'deviant behaviour' is used non-specifically to indicate any kind of behaviour, whether pathological or otherwise, that is not usual or within the limits of recognized normality in the society concerned.

In every society extremes of insanity are recognized; i.e. at some point in the range of possible human behaviour from the normal to the abnormal, the society comes to regard the individual as insane, or whatever may be the synonym for this concept. However, the attitude of society to other behaviour, which is not as abnormal as that regarded as insane, differs very much from society to society. For example, society may recognize certain individuals as being eccentric; and others as being dis-

---

[1] Theocratic guilt is a sentiment connected with the individual's observance of Divine law and his consciousness of transgression.

[2] See Rümke (1953a, p. 137): 'It appears to me to be useful to make a distinction between infantile and mature guilt . . .' and (ibid. p. 140): 'In this connection I would draw attention to the remarkable fact that infantile guilt may originate from anxiety over the possible loss of love, whereas the basis of a mature sense of guilt may be a feeling of deficiency in loving.'

turbed; still others may be regarded as vulnerable, in the sense that if things go wrong with them they may show disturbed behaviour. Again, similar items of behaviour are recognized by society as harmless in some instances and dangerous or noxious in others. It seems likely that the attitude to deviant behaviour in a society depends to some extent upon the degree of determinism in the beliefs of the people. When, for example, psychiatric theories are in conflict with a position of psychic predestination in religion, there may be a wide disparity between the 'mental health' view and the religious view, not only of abnormal behaviour but of what ought to be done about it.

The discussion ranged over various ways evolved by societies in order to deal with the eccentrics, the vulnerable, and the disturbed among their people. It may be that a society shelters or, perhaps, persecutes those who are regarded as insane, or alternatively they may be left alone as long as their behaviour is judged innocuous. Similarly, social attitudes vary towards those innocuous eccentrics who withdraw from active responsibility and participation in community life. They may be ignored, tolerated and allowed to live their own lives, assisted in their way of life, subjected to attempts at rehabilitation, excluded from society by removal into an institution, or neglected and, in extreme instances, allowed to die from starvation.

Examples of social institutions that shelter eccentric, vulnerable, and disturbed members of the community have been found in many societies and at many periods of history. In the Christendom of the Middle Ages, religious communities played a very important function in this regard, both giving shelter to such people by design and also inadvertently by finding a way of life for many eccentric individuals. Religious communities in many parts of the world and of many religions are still serving this function.

In many rural societies it is characteristic of village life that a small number of eccentrics are sheltered by the community and not only left undisturbed, but also may be found useful employment within their limitations. Among the industrialized countries of the West it is commonly found that large organizations also will find employment for a few individuals who are regarded by everyone as being not quite socially responsible, but who are tolerated as members of the community for various reasons. At another level, it is also found that universities, libraries, museums, and some other places with highly specialized functions can include incidentally a few eccentric people, who thus can contribute out of their strength, without being required to compete in society when their weaknesses might disqualify them.

There have been innumerable examples of the more passive toleration of eccentric, vulnerable, and disturbed people in society. A common solution is more or less organized vagrancy – the 'tramp' or 'hobo'. In sixteenth-century England the Poor Law provided food and shelter for vagrants in return for a prescribed amount of work. In Western countries generally it is usual for Authority to turn a blind eye to vagrancy, provided that laws are not openly flouted. In Islam religious mendicants are tolerated by society and allowed to live in freedom. In India, too, religious mendicancy may be a 'shelter', and a particularly interesting example is that of the Senyussi, people who have taken to the jungle for a variety of reasons and live there an unorganized existence outside the pale of society but supported by the religious feeling of neighbouring communities.

The attitude of society to psychotic behaviour and the treatment given to eccentric, vulnerable, and disturbed members are important considerations in any programme which includes among its aims that of getting psychiatric treatment started early, and which may raise the possibility of removal of the individual from the community. When psychiatric work is introduced into a community where little has been done previously, there may be some danger of invading the sheltered position of the people whom it is intended to help, without compensating them for what they have lost. When some interference in the life of an individual is contemplated in the supposed interests of mental health, it seems that at least the true interests of the individual demand some investigation of the degree to which his eccentricity contributes to his social conduct and his work performance. It is also important to estimate the amount of harm that his eccentricity will do to his work and to his relations with his colleagues and neighbours. It is possible to conceive of many positions in literary and cultural life as suggested above, which may be held by very eccentric people without harm, but with contributions which might not have been made by more 'normal' people.

In a community where, in the past, innocuous eccentrics have been tolerated as religious mendicants, their ascertainment as psychotic and removal to a newly built hospital, though felt to be desirable from a psychiatric point of view, might be the reverse of helpful in terms of the individual's longer-term interests.

Our discussion also touched upon the degree to which both public and psychiatric attitudes to eccentric behaviour may also be reflected in morbidity statistics. For example, study of the published statistics in Great Britain ·and other countries too, indicates areas where the mental-hospital rate is about half that of the country as a whole, and other areas, not markedly dissimilar, where the mental-hospital rate is double. This might lead to the conclusion that the actual mental-illness rate differs very widely from the population average in these areas. But there is insufficient evidence to justify any such conclusion, and a number of other factors need consideration. First, there is the public attitude to psychotic behaviour; where there is tolerance of and capacity to shelter the psychotic individual, there may be no great impetus to secure hospital treatment for the sufferer, and in this event the recognized incidence of disorder would be low. Second, the public attitude to the mental hospitals concerned makes a difference to the use that is made of the hospital by the community. There are class differences in attitude also, both to hospitals and to psychotic behaviour. In those regions in which the mental hospitals have an indifferent reputation with the public, there is naturally a tendency to conceal cases of psychosis. Another region may enjoy an efficient mental-hospital service which commands a good reputation and has the trust of the population, with the natural result of a tendency to seek treatment earlier by people of many classes.

It will be generally agreed that the subject of attitude towards psychotic behaviour requires a great deal more research.

Ecstasy

Another problem in the introduction of mental health work to a community where none has existed before is the attitude of the community to experience felt to be ecstatic by the members of the group, whether the experience be of a religious or secular nature. There may be wide variations between different cultures in public attitude towards ecstatic experience, and an even wider gulf may exist between the public attitude and the psychiatric point of view. Where the psychiatric view differs widely from the public attitude, difficult problems can arise, also, from the too rapid and uncritical acceptance of psychiatric ideas among the lay population, which it is possible, might be more dangerous than helpful to the community. It is desirable that new thinking on this subject be digested and reformulated in indigenous terms and in local languages before it becomes general property, otherwise many problems may be encountered that might never have arisen. It is valuable, therefore, to explore the existing attitudes of the community to ecstatic experience and relate these to the attitudes of the mental health specialists who work there.

The subject is further complicated by the possibility that in considering the nature of psychosensorial experiences there may be a failure to distinguish between the phenomenon or symptom, and its content.

In the course of our discussion about human behaviour, it was remarked that the range both of experiencing and of expressing mechanisms is small and therefore that the same psychological processes are manifested in different behavioural phenomena. This may lead psychiatrists, for example, to take a 'psychiatric view' of certain phenomena otherwise regarded as manifestations of religion. An illustration of this is found in Franz Alexander's writing (1931) on Hindu mysticism, which he is inclined to regard as a form of artificial catatonic behaviour.

The usual psychiatric view of the sensory side of ecstatic experience is that the phenomenon is of the order of hallucination, that is to say, a psychological process which, though it may be pathological, is not necessarily so. There are many conditions in which hallucinations may be experienced and which carry no suggestion of psychological illness. For example, in 'twilight states' between waking and sleeping, especially under conditions of fatigue or bodily stress, such as high fever, it is quite common for people to have hallucinatory experiences. Alcohol and many drugs can produce similar results. Eidetic imagery, which is normal among many children, has frequently been found to persist into adult life; and it could be argued that the reporting of mystical manifestations or even, conceivably, of flying saucers, may owe something to the persistence of eidetic imagery in an individual with a strong emotional drive to have the experience in question.

There are many cases recorded of communities where ecstatic experiences are accepted as the normal and even, to some extent, institutionalized. An illustration of this is the case of the North American plains Indians, among whom visions and ecstatic experiences are a recognized part of life, but subject to cultural rules. That is to say, there is an accepted convention as to what constitutes a 'right' vision that will be acceptable to the community. An individual having a vision that is unacceptable will be ignored and the vision given no significance by other members of the tribe (see Lowie, 1935).

The case of Socrates is often quoted in this connection; he

is reported to have had some behavioural idiosyncrasies, the nature of which cannot be definitely determined. For example, he accepted the guidance of his *daimonion,* whose 'voice' he heard on many occasions. From a psychiatric point of view, the phenomenon resembles schizophrenic auditory hallucinations.

The case of Jeanne d'Arc is another illustration. It is possible, if one were to regard her behaviour from an exclusively psychiatric point of view, to conclude that hers was a case of transvestism with hallucinations. On this evidence alone, one might claim that she was psychotic. However, the possibility must be considered that her experiences might have had other, including transcendental, origins.

The assessment of individual ecstatic experience by the community as a whole will take two main forms, and these forms are also used by psychiatrists. The first is by the use of criteria such as 'style of behaviour', consistency of behaviour, and reality orientation; and the second is the assessment of behaviour by the consequences to which the experience leads. In many Western countries the determination of the presence of 'insanity' is a matter of legal decision, and it is noteworthy that the main criterion used is not the experience itself but its consequences. In the canonization of Saints in the Roman Catholic church, one of the main criteria used, likewise, is the consequence of the mystical experience and not the experience itself. What appear to be mystical experiences, therefore, can have different styles of interpretation, in terms of pathology and of religious experience, respectively.

In the considering of the canonization of Saints the question of hysterical phenomena is very often a source of considerable difficulty requiring exhaustive investigation. The case of Theresa Neumann illustrated this. Her mystical experiences have been very carefully investigated by a number of commissions including psychiatrists. The conclusion has tended towards the opinion that it is possible that she could have had her experiences by naturalistic means, i.e. that to some extent they may have been derived from hysterical mechanisms. The result has been that she may be accepted as a holy person but it is conceded that her experiences could have had a natural explanation (see Siwek, 1953).

The criterion of the consequences of ecstatic experiences may become obscure and complicated in the case of known recoveries from advanced somatic illness subsequent to mystical experience or faith-healing. A good deal more information is required on this point; but we would agree that the individual's acceptance of his fate and identification with a transcendental motive can influence recovery from an illness.

These observations do not entirely resolve the questions raised by community phenomena which can be regarded variously as hysteria or as ecstasy. Even the most extreme and apparently spontaneous ecstatic behaviour may be very severely regulated by society. So in Bali, there are appropriate occasions and appropriate individuals for a trance ceremony. Those who fall into trances prematurely, or inappropriately in other ways, are simply requested to absent themselves from the ceremonies. Thus a distinction should be drawn between the psychological validity of the trance state, and the ceremonial efficacy (see Bateson & Mead, 1942; Belo, 1960).

The public attitude to ecstatic experiences and related phenomena is of practical importance, for example, in the selection of people who are entering public positions. Perhaps the most relevant instance is that of candidates for religious missions or the religious ministry, and it appears that a great deal more knowledge is needed before selection methods will become reliable in this field.

Mental Health Assumptions and Implications

Relationships within the Family

One fairly widespread view has it that neurosis is almost synonymous with failure in development, i.e. that something goes wrong; which among other after-effects disturbs the relationship between the individual and the group. Generally, exact knowledge in this field is slight. We know little of the effect of single patterns of stress in the early relationships of young children, with the exception of a limited number of cases of stress acting in a specific context at a specific time. An example of the latter is that of total neglect in infancy, some of the consequences of which have been studied by Bowlby (1951) and others, who have set out some of the evidence established about the causal connection between disturbances of the mother and child relationship in early infancy and disturbances in mental health later. Generally speaking it must be admitted that evidence in this field is still incomplete and often conflicting, for although most clinicians would regard the situation as sufficiently proven to justify the exercise of care to prevent infants being deprived of normal maternal nurture, this does not constitute a scientific proof.

Our problem here is to consider to what extent observations about family relationship can or cannot be extrapolated from one culture to another without clarification and adaptation. There are many questions which might be asked; for example, is there any significant difference between the emotional attitudes of Buddhist mothers and Western Christian mothers, respectively, towards their infants? In Buddhism there is a high value set on non-attachment; does a mother in a Buddhist culture form a similar intensity of attachment to her infant to that which is standard in the West? If it were a fact that Buddhist mothers were less emotionally attached to their infants than Western Christian mothers, would it not be logical to suppose that mother-child separation would have a less serious effect in the former case? Would the phenomenon of non-attachment result in the formation of relationships in the family at a lower degree of emotional tension, as it were; and if so has this any association with the peacefulness or serenity which is sometimes attributed by Westerners to the Buddhist character pattern? These are complicated issues and their discussion would involve consideration of the differences to be found in relationships within the extended family system as compared with the nuclear family.

Attitudes of Social Superiority and Inferiority

Attitudes of social superiority and inferiority are related to the value set on human beings in a society. Our view is that the assumption of an attitude of superiority by one social group towards another is not conducive to the mental health of either group. Further, in our view, it would be unsafe to assume that any group of people that had been in contact with another group that defined itself as superior could be completely happy with their situation.

In the Southern States of the U.S.A. the opinion is often stated that the Negro is contented so long as he remains in a position of relative peonage. Research has shown that this is not true. Scientific studies have been made of the attitudes of Negro children towards their own skin colour and, whether in the North or the South of the U.S.A., they tend to show disturbed reactions, to be aware of their inferior hierarchical position and to react to it rather violently (see Clark, 1955).

It appears to us that the members of a group of individuals who remain contented while they are in an inferior position in society fail to satisfy some of the important criteria of mental health. We would like also to question the state of mental health of the 'superior' group in that society.

According to a Western-trained Indian psychiatrist, the Hindu caste system, at a time when it was not seriously challenged, was an exception to the principle enunciated above; the people in inferior castes accepted their inferior position as Karma, and perhaps they were neither contented nor discontented with their lot, for their religion set a high value on acceptance. This argument needs to be considered critically lest it represents no more than a rationalization or perhaps a repression of tendencies operating against the established system. Moreover, it could be argued that acceptance of the social system in this case is not evidence of mental health in that society, on the grounds that lower-caste, and particularly out-caste, society in the Hindu system does not provide for the complete range of human potentialities. This is one of the criteria that we have adopted of mental health in a society.

Independence and Maturity

It is hardly possible to conceive of a completely independent person in any culture, for the concept of complete independence of an individual involves the notion of an infinite concept of the self, and is philosophically unacceptable. However, just as dependence is characteristic of infancy, so an increasing degree of independence is characteristic of the normal course of maturation. Questions that might be studied with advantage are: whether the mature individual is regarded similarly or differently in various cultures; to what extent maturity involves a concept of personal independence; and how far the necessity for the individual to stand on his own feet is harmonized with the dependence upon others that the individual will have in every society. Another field of inquiry can be outlined by a specific illustration: there is a difference between the kind of maturity expected of a young person in Western society when getting married, and the quality of maturity that goes with the dependence of young married couples on the extended Indian or Chinese family.[1]

[1] It is worthy of note that in North America, and to a less extent in Western Europe, changes are occurring currently in attitudes to the marriage of young people while still dependent. Thus, it is now common for marriages to take place during the college or vocational training period; but in these cases, still a small minority, only the parents of the couple will be involved in their support, and it will not be the responsibility of the family as a whole.

One aspect of the concept of maturity worth further consideration is that of the meaningfulness of the ideology to the people concerned; or what might be described as the saturation of society by religion. For example; to what extent does the religion or ideology involve the masses, in addition to those professionally concerned; and, to what extent is it a living centre of life or an outward cultural form that merely serves as a framework?

These questions might be studied through the ethical aspirations of the society and its ways of dealing with guilt, sin, shame, etc. What level of aspiration is expected of the individual? To what extent in the culture is it possible for a mentally-ill person to adapt to cultural behaviour at a low level? Are the expectations of the society such that an individual can adapt at a low level without being subjected to undue stress? (See also p. 77.)

Behind all these questions it is important to consider the individual's wants and how near can he get to attaining his wants in his own society; what desires the society stimulates in the individual; and whether it promotes the satisfaction of the desires it stimulates, or not (see also p. 86). This leads to discussion of the position of the reformer *vis-à-vis* society; and to a further question, is it better for the society to have in it a number of potential Socrates who are unsatisfied; or the mass of the people who are satisfied?

Anthropological studies have shown that in Samoa the people learned to make limited demands, which the culture met. The majority of the people appeared satisfied but it seems that the more intense people and the more imaginative dreamers in that society contributed little. This is a further illustration of the point made in a previous discussion that social adaptation is not necessarily equivalent to mental health. One aspect of mal-adaptation is that of the unsatisfied dreamer. Dreams for the future in a society in which they can be satisfied may be conducive to mental health both of the individual and of the society, and might appear there as productive imagination. Dreams in a society in which they could not be realized are not conducive to mental health and might appear there as unproductive fantasy.

Adaptation

The history of social institutions shows periods of growth, flexibility, integrated stability, stagnation, rigidity, and disintegration. There may be some tendency to mistake the changes which occur in individuals and institutions alike, during the different phases of their existence, with a capacity for adaptation that is supposed to indicate mental health. Thus we need to explore further the extent to which social adaptation is relevant to the concept of mental health.

It appears to us that capacity for adaptation is in some senses an ambitropic quality. It has been agreed that capacity for adaptation is an important component of mental health; but mental ill-health also can be marked by the individual's adaptation to his illness. This can be illustrated by the case of the psychotic patient who becomes identified with his pathological mental experiences. The behaviour of the patient, however bizarre it may seem, may represent a particular kind of adaptation to the new state of affairs. However, the psychotic patient does not usually retain his full capacity for adaptation to external reality (nor to his internal world). In comparison with the psychotic, the psychoneurotic patient, who may retain insight, retains a greater capacity for adapting to external reality, but shows less capacity for adapting to his pathological mental experience. Therefore, a main difference between these two classes of patient is the direction in which they show adaptive capacity.

A parallel might be drawn also with the case of disturbances arising in social institutions, and in which analogous variations in individual capacity for adaptation may be seen.

Another formulation of a similar nature has been made by a Western-trained psychiatrist who has described mental health as a dynamic equilibrium of the personality. The forces maintaining the equilibrium are operating at different levels of the living organism, from a level less differentiated than that of the cell, as in the maintenance of tissue fluid balances, to the level of complex mental processes.

Dynamic equilibrium, it is suggested, is made up of the interaction of two basic characteristic tendencies: that to maintain constancy and perpetuate life; and that which leads in the direction of differentiation, growth, and change. This interaction calls for regulating mechanisms. Thus, dynamic equilibrium, in the sense employed here, implies a continuous integration of these opposing tendencies.

Trends towards mental health will be in the direction of the resolution of tension, and of evolution in relation to the environment. Unresolved tensions may lead to anxiety, and various pathological phenomena may appear, of which undue aggression or regression are examples.

If adaptation can lead in the direction both of mental health and of mental ill-health, it is important to recognize which direction the process is taking. This is a broad field of study and has been illustrated above in the discussion touching upon individual and group behaviour of a regressive quality that may indicate adaptive trends in the direction of ill-health.

A paradoxical situation sometimes arises when a psychiatrist helps an individual to enlarge his ability to adapt to his own society. On occasion the adaptation towards which the psychiatrist attempts to help the individual appears to the observer to lead to the direction of mental ill-health. An example of this is the release of repressed aggression which may sometimes result in a phase of more disturbed behaviour – the antithesis of improvement in the eyes of the outside observer.

Mental Health in Changing Societies

We need to consider further the concept of mental health in its relation to change in society. We have seen that complete harmony, that is, living in social adjustment, is not in itself evidence óf mental health. It is clear that the importance to an individual of a capacity to adapt will vary according to the degree to which change is happening in the culture. If the culture itself is not changing, or is changing at a very slow rate, conformity with the culture is a rule of life and in such conditions a specific and separable concept of mental health is obscure. If the culture is strictly unchanging (though this is a theoretical rather than a practical consideration) conformity is the highest value and no separable concept of mental health is possible.

On the other hand, if the culture is itself changing, then adjustment to the culture will be impossible unless the individual is changing too, and, also, in this situation, mental health can have some meaning as an aspiration. It appears that the mental health of the individual will depend upon the relationship maintained between individual and institutional change.

In the WFMH Study No. I on 'Identity' we have considered the concept of 'identity strength'. In Section IX, pages 34–38, the importance of continuity, coherence, and flexibility of identity was discussed. It was suggested that a tendency exists in the personality towards integration, having a general managerial function, and which we defined as 'identity strength'.

Identity strength lies also in the relation of the past to the present and to the future. This does not imply that, for identity strength, behaviour must necessarily be totally consistent, for there are many ways in which temporary changes in behaviour involving abrogation of responsibility and, to a greater or lesser extent a break in identity, are formalized and made acceptable in society. Such ways may include fatigue, minor infection, or headache on the one hand, and a wide range of those phenomena which may extend as far as states of dissociation and trances on the other. The mental health concern in this area will be with the promotion of identity strength and the prevention of excessive strain on identity formation. In the latter respect it is possible that a socially acceptable way of easing tension, such as a psychosomatic symptom, may itself ultimately increase the difficulties of the individual if it should interfere with reality orientation.

Mental Health and Value Systems

Definition of a Universal Phenomenon

A universal phenomenon, as defined here, is one that prevails in all known societies even though there may be many variations in form and content. We would like to pose the question whether it is possible to find any attitudes that are universally regarded as mentally healthy. Our object would be to find some statements that have wide cross-cultural applicability.

In the discussion it was suggested that every known culture values human beings; human group relationships; and makes value judgments about certain states of human beings, such as birth, infancy, maturation, reproduction, physical maladies and anomalies, old age, and death. Our problem is to find out how such matters are regarded in different cultures. It is possible to say that all cultures have values, but not to say, for example, that in all cultures newborn infants are valued, for in some only those infants who have been selected for survival are valued, or only those infants who have demonstrated their ability to survive. Similarly hunger, thirst, fatigue, and fear are recognized in all known cultures, and placed on a value scale, but they may be regarded in many different ways, as tests of fortitude, for example, or something to be avoided at all costs. Again, dependency may be an attitude to be cultivated or overcome; responsibility something to strive for or to avoid.

We may recognize the existence of universal human phenomena such as the care of infants, and the provision of food for children, teaching and learning of language, the development of a sense of orientation and identity, the ability to handle symbolism, the recognition of some form of relationship to the universe. No society is known in which the killing of a member of the group is not judged differently from the killing of a non-group member. Primary incest taboos exist in all cultures.

We find everywhere culturally characteristic attitudes towards privacy and property; and universal group phenomena, such as sibling rivalry, the inhibition of aggressiveness in society, the making of a distinction between one's own group and a stranger, and hospitality. There are universal institutions such as family, religious and political structures; and universal psychological principles, such as repression, projection, identification, and memory. The members of all known cultures have characteristic attitudes towards fate – to the past, the present, and the future.

Humanity universally has gone beyond the pleasure principle into instinct modification and into the spheres of other value systems (including metaphysics, philosophy, and religion). All human beings have systems of evaluation.

It is suggested that universal phenomena in the field of our discussion might be organized into five classes: (i) events, (ii) experiences, (iii) institutional or cultural features, (iv) psychological processes, and (v) conceptions. However, both this classification and the statement made above that certain events are noted, certain conditions recognized, and certain restrictions observed in all cultures, are only first steps in the establishment of any cross-culturally applicable definition of mental health. It may be expected that the search for examples of attitudes that are universally regarded as mentally healthy will have to be conducted in a higher order of abstraction, in which the relationships among the various values within a culture are given due weight.

Growth and Development

There is probably a growing recognition of the likelihood that appropriate loving treatment as a baby is a *conditio sine qua non* of a child's later capacity for human understanding and affective development. There is as yet not enough scientific evidence to make this a biological law, and it is known that not every mother is able to love her baby in the same way; however, it is a valid generalization to state that all cultures take a moral attitude towards the relationships between parents and children.

Clinical evidence suggests that there are some babies who,

for one reason or another, are incapable of responding to maternal love in such a way as to make love a normal reciprocal state. Whereas in the case of some babies this is due to a passive state of lack of response, in the case of others a more definite failure to relate is apparent. Thus there are potential causes in the case of both parties, the mother and the child, for the failure of love to develop. This state of affairs is borne out by experience, which shows that mutual love does not develop universally between mother and baby.

No one who has religious conceptions finds it practicable to make an absolute distinction between certain basic living processes which belong to the human being as such, e.g. a particular baby's capacity to develop love with its mother; and religious conceptions, e.g. love, in the abstract. To the religious person, both are part of the human being's life, not only in relation to his fellows, but also in relation to God. It appears to us that though a gap will often appear between the intellectual and emotional growth of individuals, religious people universally will believe that things mental, spiritual, and physical all belong together, that the whole thing is a living process. The belief that living is a unified process will not be confined to religious people, of course.

Attainment of developmental goals in a balanced way is sometimes thought of as maturity, which, as we have already discussed, is not synonymous with mental health. The latter has different criteria in different situations and at different stages of life. For example, a person in an isolated, primitive society is mentally healthy in so far as he can meet the demands which come to him, but as wider social life opens out to him the demands become greater; if he is to continue to be mentally healthy he must show an adaptability and an elasticity of response to growing demand. Mental health alone is not the aspiration, but makes possible the fulfilment of the aspiration.

Balance and Development

In the daily life of human beings there is a need for participation in the outer world to be balanced by what is done with experiential material internally and then given out again. If, like the Samoans, people take in little and give out little, there can still be a balance. On the other hand, an individual might find the impact of the outer world so rich that he could not deal with it, or he might have an inner world too rich to deal with; in both cases there would be lack of balance (see Alexander & Ross, 1952).

Growth is a universal phenomenon and it is an inherent part of the growing process that there will be some instability. In the presence of development from one phase to another the existing order will often become unstable, perhaps disintegrate, and then be replaced by something new.

> This might be illustrated from the process of weaning, in which well-established feeding habits of the baby are broken down and become disintegrated in the process of establishing new ways of feeding. The instability which accompanies the breaking down of an old way of life cannot strictly be regarded as ill-health, and it is part of the process of growth. It, rather, constitutes an obstacle which, if successfully negotiated by the mother and child, will lead the latter to a higher level of maturity.

Such periods of instability heralding new development might be described as productive disintegration (see Rümke, 1953b).

SUMMARY

Attempts to define mental health have progressively laid greater emphasis on more 'positive' factors. Current approaches show concern with the internal balance of the individual, the quality of the relationships between the individual and others, and the attitudes of groups to these relationships.

The discussion deals with a number of questions; for example, does the concept of mental health and its derivative behaviour mean different things to different people? What is the relation between such matters as social approval, happiness, the concept of goodness, adaptability, conformity, maturity, social harmony, contentment, belief in God, etc., and the concept of mental health? Adaptability is a good case in point. Societies differ in the degree to which they permit variations in the adaptation of the individual. Is the relationship between adaptability and mental health affected by such variations? What is the mental health position of the individual who has adapted to the ethos of a small religious cult that is at variance with society at large? Given that adaptability is important for mental health, is it possible that adaptability can also lead in the direction of mental illness, as in the case of the psychotic individual who becomes identified with his pathological processes. To what extent does lack of adaptability contribute to social stresses that may impair mental health?

Is deviant behaviour a sign of poor mental health? Since social attitudes tend to change, the criterion of social acceptance of behaviour is unreliable. For what degree of deviant behaviour is the individual held responsible by society? Practically all cultures recognize a certain degree of disturbance of behaviour as irresponsible, but in all societies we know people will insist upon individual responsibility for some aspects of deviant behaviour, and term it wrong.

To what extent do societies differ in their toleration of deviant behaviour and make provision for eccentric and deviant individuals in the structure of society? The subject of ecstatic behaviour is a field in which religious and 'mental health' attitudes overlap and frequently conflict.

In spite of the many assumptions that are made about the components of mental health, exact knowledge in this field is insufficient. Is it possible to go further than general statements such as, 'babies need their mothers' love and care'?

Among the questions discussed as relevant to the concept of mental health in society are the following: Is the value set upon interpersonal affect within the family the same in the case of all religions? Is mental health compatible with the acceptance of either an inferior or a superior position in society, whether in regard to individual or to group relationships? How do concepts of independence, maturity, and so on vary in different cultural patterns? Are there variations in the degree that the ordinary person in society is involved in the religion or ideology of the group, or in levels of aspiration demanded of the individual? Are there societies in which individuals can adapt at a low level without stress? To what extent do societies promote, allow, or forbid the satisfaction of all the desires that are stimulated by life in that society?

Mental health can be regarded in one sense as a dynamic equilibrium between constancy on the one hand and differentiation, growth, and change on the other.

Mental health work must be carefully attuned to change that is taking place in the society concerned. To what extent is identity strength, its continuity, coherence, and flexibility, important in mental health? Is it possible for identity strength, and therefore mental health, to be preserved if temporary changes of behaviour, such as psychosomatic symptomatology and dissociative phenomena, are permitted without social penalty in times of stress?

Finally, certain universal values concerned with human life and attitudes are discussed. For example, development, which is a universal biological phenomenon, presupposes the disappearance of an existing order and its replacement by something new. How can the instability that heralds a new development be distinguished from that which precedes disintegration?

CHAPTER 2

Relevant Material
from Various Religions and Ideologies

INTRODUCTION

THE NEXT step is to present material that throws light upon
variations relevant to our subject that exist among different
religions and ideologies. Some of the selections that are given
below have been taken from the two conferences on religion and
mental health that have been held in connection with this project, and others have been gleaned from discussion in committee
and from reading.

In general, material has been selected solely because of its
inherent interest; few of the selections are authoritative or representative, and none is exhaustive. Their main significance is that
of a number of examples of interesting phenomena as seen in
various cultural settings by certain highly qualified individuals.
We do not presume to judge the accuracy or objectivity of these
statements which we have reproduced. In most cases the cultural
examples that we have taken have been presented by people
coming from the culture concerned and although they may not
be representative of widespread phenomena they can at least be
said to have occurred.

The conference that was held in New York identified a number of contrasting tendencies in human behaviour, including
autonomy and dependence; understanding by the individual and
acceptance of authority; consistency and flexibility; temporal,
this-worldly, and eternal, other-worldly; natural good versus

natural evil; necessity for internal change and necessity for external change; individual and group. Although for the want of a better term we have referred to them as contrasting tendencies, they need not be regarded as dichotomous or mutually exclusive. It is hoped that the examples in the text will illustrate the complexity of these concepts.

VARIATIONS IN VALUE SYSTEMS

An Islamic Concept of Mental Health

We were informed by a Sudanese psychiatrist, who is widely acquainted with Western thought, that in the Sudan the definition of mental health has been made difficult by changes that have occurred in the people's conception of the aspirations bound up with their pursuit of health. The first mention of the term mental health as distinct from mental disorder that can be found in the Islamic culture was that by a Persian mystic, Jalal el Din Mohamed Assaad (died 1502), but the term remained unused. It appears to have been a theoretical curiosity and its preventive connotation was not recognized.

In many parts of the Islamic world, concepts of human adjustment and of the interaction of good with evil have been changing, and some things that were earlier thought to have contributed positively and constructively to human good are nowadays regarded as being harmful. In such changes, utility appears to be an important influence.

In the Sudan itself, we understand, thinkers on these subjects regard the subject of mental health as extremely complex, concepts are changing and different developments are occurring in different parts of the country.

Examples can be found in the Islamic world of institutions that have existed for centuries without being regarded as incompatible with mental health in so far as any such concept existed, until with the more recent impact of Western cultures attitudes have changed. For example, polygamy has in general been regarded by the Sudanese as good, and this, we are informed, is because of the survival value ascribed to polygamy for the communities that practise it. In a nomadic culture, it is said, when man-power becomes a crucial issue in survival and where child-mortality rates are high, polygamy is almost a biological necessity. But as a result of sweeping changes due to alterations in health conditions and economic and social circumstances, it is now becoming common in the Sudan for polygamy to be regarded as incompatible with mental health. The significance of this, as an example of the operation of the Moslem concept of utility as an important value, will be discussed further on page 155.

The validity of many other customs and usages, not only in Islam but in other cultures and societies, is now being questioned, although for centuries they may have been regarded by the community as beneficial. As attitudes change, such customs tend to be regarded as obstacles in the path of the development of the culture, but notions of this kind are necessarily relative to time and space, and to historical development. It may be concluded that, except in a very limited sense and as applied to the unities of time, place, and the human beings involved, there is no such thing, strictly, as compatibility or incompatibility with mental health. Customs or practices regarded as compatible with mental health today may be considered harmful tomorrow.

Sikhism – the Attainable Ideal

An important concept among the Sikhs is that of the 'Ideal Sikh' which is an attainable ideal, expressed in terms of human behaviour, and is quite distinct from any concept of 'God'. A Sikh may have anxiety because he is not living up to the ideal, but whatever his conduct, he cannot be denied the security of his group allegiance and of his position in the family. Baptism, which is of adults only, is also open to him as a reaffirmation of his principles and a public declaration that wins him considerable prestige.

A Confucian Ideal Attribute

The notion permeates much Confucian writing that man is

perfectible – that is, that everyone can move towards the ideal. In the Confucian case, however, the ideal is defined in much more abstract terms, and in descriptions of role behaviour rather than of human attributes. Responsibility for moving towards the ideal is placed both on the parents and on the person himself. It is of interest in this connection, that among the orthodox Confucian Chinese, we understand, when it is felt that a young man's behaviour should be criticized this is not done direct, but to the parents, instead.

Confucian Values

A Western-trained Chinese psychiatrist, speaking about Confucian values, made a distinction between good as defined in abstractions and as in the description of roles. Confucius, while stressing roles (i.e. human relationships) also talked of Benevolence, Justice, Propriety, and Wisdom. He explained the latter in terms of social relationships. A conscience able to function well in all situations must rest, as far as possible, on abstractions; but for practical purposes abstractions must be defined in concrete terms, otherwise they provide no guidance.

It appears logical to suppose that in a patriarchal culture reinforced by the images of numerous ancestor-figures, the formation of the superego, to use the psycho-analytical term, will be powerful. Equally a culture belief in an all-knowing, punishing, or rewarding God also tends to strengthen the superego; but in Confucianism such a concept of an anthropomorphic God is weak.

Our informant on Confucian attitudes added that the notion that the mature superego is able to depart from the fierce and primitive talion principle of an eye for an eye is embodied in the Confucian principle of harmony and the Golden Mean. This principle takes into account the needs of the individual and the demands of society, and harmonizes them; it does not adhere to a rigid legalistic approach to wrong-doing. The attitude of Confucius is well expressed in

Mental Health and Value Systems

the phrases: 'Requite evil with justice.' 'In sentencing a man have pity on him and do not be proud of it.'

We are informed that Confucius did not seek supernatural authority for his ethics, but ascribed them to the Emperors Yao and Shun who were culture heroes, and as such possessed a certain numinous quality. This is in line with the historical fact that the Chinese people always regarded themselves as having the right to revolt against the Emperor if things went badly wrong. He was subject to moral judgment and if he failed it was held that the mandate of Heaven had been withdrawn from him.

A Remark on Values in Russia

A social scientist studying the value systems of modern Soviet Russia remarked that history is, as it were, taking the place of God in Soviet Russia, where a new kind of transcendental religion is evolving. In the amnesty which can be given to deviant individuals after admission of error and restoration to the group there is something of the kind of experience of absolution familiar in Christian practice. It can hardly be believed that the viability of the whole Soviet system is the viability of materialistic atheism, alone.

Non-material Value System

A Roman Catholic priest and psychologist said that if the individual with whom a mental health worker was dealing believed in something other than the material universe, and conceived himself to be related to this non-material reality, the mental health worker should bear this attitude of the patient constantly in mind.

This situation occasionally becomes an important feature of a case. It can be illustrated by the dilemma of a patient for whom a significant scale of values exists, related to his concept of non-material reality, and who may be faced with the choice or not of a course of action designed to lead to a cure of his condition that is not consonant with his personal value system. It makes no difference to the objective importance of this dilemma to the patient if the mental health worker accepts for himself or rejects the values that are significant to the patient. As an extreme example, the choice might lie between achieving a cure and jeopardizing the patient's relation with God. It is an important question whether it is the duty of the psychiatrist to accept the patient's valuation, when that is so, that his religion or existing scale of values is more important to him even than a cure; or whether the psychiatrist's duty is to remain exclusively scientific, and work for the cure of the patient, regardless of the effect upon his religion.

Hinduism – the Holy Man

A Western-trained Indian psychiatrist spoke of the seventeen million or so Senyussi in India, who live as religious mendicants, mostly in the forests and open country, and who wear a minimum of clothing. He remarked that the rest of the population regard them, on the whole, as religious people who have seen God, who have renounced the things of the flesh, and they have the popular reputation of being very happy in their life. But from the medical or psychiatric point of view many of them are schizophrenics or other unstable characters who avoid responsibility or who can accept no form of work or who are mentally defective. Some of them are not unlike the severe neurotics of the West but, unlike the latter, the Senyussi, as an alternative to social collapse or even suicide, become religious mendicants. In their lucid intervals they may behave rationally but at other times their mood may be more ecstatic, in that visions of God are frequently reported. One such man had epilepsy and his disciples noted down his sayings during a pre-epileptic aura, claiming he had had a visitation from God (see also p. 97).

Our informant also spoke of another Indian group, the Hata Yogins, who often show eccentric social behaviour; for instance they may spend long periods standing on one leg, or sleep on a bed of nails, or remain mute. To the population, to stand on one leg may be a sign of holiness and the man may be offered food and clothing and even worshipped; but to the psychiatrist such behaviour is more likely to be taken as a sign of psychosis.

The ordinary people of the local communities believe, on the whole, that these men are happy; and indeed they often believe that because the Hata Yogins have renounced the joys of the flesh and because their attitude to wealth, comforts, drink, food, and sex is different from that of ordinary people, mental happiness therefore lies in renouncing the desires of the flesh. Asceticism as practised by the Hata Yogins may then become the general criterion of perfect mental health, a criterion that is strengthened by the impression that those who practise it are apparently unaffected by any changes happening in the world. But more objectively speaking and certainly from the point of view of a psychiatrist, whether Eastern or Western, the Hata Yogins are living in a world of fantasy, and in many ways they resemble those patients in mental hospitals in Western countries who also may seem to be quite happy and to have become identified with their fantasy worlds.

Even if it were conceded as a fact that ordinary Indian people think that the asceticism of the Hata Yogins is a sign of mental health, there would still be a further question to concern us, which is what Indian doctors and psychiatrists think about the mental health of these people. This question needs examining with great care, because some form of asceticism may fit naturally into the context of a man's way of life and his surroundings. The psychiatrist must be careful to distinguish between such asceticism and behaviour that may appear to be similar but is in fact due to something else, more of the order of self-punishment (see p. 101).

A note on Imagery and Religious Concepts

A practising pastoral psychologist has reflected upon some possible effects of the predominance of visual imagery among some people, and of auditory imagery among others. People with different types of imagery might respond differently to leadership, for example, and differences such as these could conceivably be important in mental health, though the effect of strong polarity in imagery will be reduced by the fact that most people seem to be mixtures of auditory and visual imagery types. If a leader of principles happened to be very strongly moved in one direction and his people tended to predominate in another, many unforeseen consequences might follow. Types of imagery might affect the theology and attitude of people to God; e.g. the Greek picture of God was strong in the dimensions of space; whereas the Hebrew idea of God was more in the temporal dimension. It would be interesting to see whether this could be related to types of imagery. It is possible that a study of symbolism might show something of the possible influence of imagery in the concept of God developed by a people, and interesting differences are provided by what we know about ancient Greek and Hebrew cultures.

RESPONSIBILITY

Society and Individual

One of the diverging tendencies to which we have referred in the introduction to this chapter concerned the nature of responsibility. In discussing here the question whether society or the individual is to be held responsible, we shall put a number of points of view that will illustrate various shifts of emphasis, but in no sense attempt an essay in comparative theology (see also p. 96).

A student of comparative religion has put forward for consideration the effects of two antithetical points of view that may be found, variously, in the major religions : (i) That man is naturally good and that if society brings him up rightly, he will go on all right. If he develops wrongly, it is not his fault. It is compatible with this view to regard his failure to adjust to society as mental ill-health, i.e. his failure becomes the fault of the society in some way. (ii) That man is not to be regarded as naturally good, and that it is possible for a man to choose evil even when there is no defect in the social system.

The question of who is held responsible – the society or the individual – is relevant to all the great religious systems.

The Confucian Attitude – Society is Responsible

We were informed by a Western-trained Chinese psychiatrist that, in principle, in Chinese tradition, when anything goes wrong it is regarded as the fault of the society and not that of the individual. If it be held that man's nature is good, it follows logically that 'society' must be blamed for wrong behaviour. But the Confucian principle is that, though man's nature is essentially good, in actual life there is no possibility of fully expressing the good without positively cultivating it. In the case of the child, the responsibility for the good rests on the parents, on teachers, and, later, on the individual as he grows up. The two parts of the basic premise that man is good but that goodness needs to be cultivated cannot be separated and they form the opening words of a child's synopsis of Confucianism. The analogy of seed and soil was actually used by Confucius, who also stressed the importance of self-cultivation by the adult.

A man might fail to cultivate his goodness and break down with anxiety. When this happens the responsibility for failure to cultivate the good would be ascribed by the traditionalist Confucian partly to society for not bringing the man up properly; and partly to the man himself on the grounds of his responsibility for cultivating his own gifts.

We examined the hypothetical case of a child who had been brought up by his parents in Confucian traditions, who had then gone to a European school and had adopted European ways, refusing to conform to the rituals of his family. It appeared to us that his family would be faced with the decision whether to regard him as delinquent because he had broken with tradition; or as ill and send him to a psychiatrist if one were available. We inquired whether it might happen that traditionalist parents might regard the boy as mentally ill, and were informed that mental illness is too strong a term to use in connection with that kind of problem in Chinese culture. If the boy did not confirm to ancestor rites or take his proper role, he would be regarded as delinquent, and the blame would be as much on the parents as on himself.

Another dimension would be entered if mental illness were to be brought into the question, and several factors have to be taken into consideration. The idea of reactive mental illness is recognized in a Confucian society, and in this respect the average lay person in Chinese society would show little difference of attitude from the rest of the world. If the boy were regarded as mentally ill by his group, i.e. grossly deviant in behaviour, there would be no question of applying moral judgment either to the boy himself or to those responsible for his education. If a minor deviation were concerned, probably the first reaction of the group would be a moral one. But the qualitative as well as the quantitative aspects of the act would have to be considered by the group.

Illness, we were told, was recognized by the ancient Chinese thinkers as derived from an imbalance of the humours (yin-yan humours) and a disorder of the five elements. An ordinary uneducated Chinese might still think along these lines today, if he considered that a medical question was involved. If he were to consider the problem morally, however, he would think along Confucian lines of the man's responsibility for cultivating his own goodness. According to our informant, Confucian writings make nothing of mental illness as such, nor of spirit possession. There is, however, a recurrent theme in Chinese Confucian thought which relates calamity to misdeeds of ancestors, and this notion might be one factor colouring the attitude towards what is recognized as illness.

Hinduism – Individual Responsibility within a Collective System

According to a Western-trained Indian Brahmin psychiatrist, the view of Hindu society is that once a man is born society owes nothing to him. A man is born into a certain estate because of something he has done in his previous life. He is given the shape of a man again in order that he may carry out a function that he has failed to carry out in the past. It is often explicit in Hindu sacred writings that the individual is born into the world with certain gifts which it is his duty to utilize to the maximum extent for the good of the world and that if he does not do so, he alone must pay the penalty, and society is not to blame. Man is supposed to have a certain amount of divine spark in him at birth, this being at its greatest among Brahmins and less in the other castes.

A Brahmin may sometimes attempt to rationalize having done something that he ought not to do when he is mentally and physically healthy, by saying that in his previous life there was a gap and what he was doing was a sort of penance. However, the rest of the community would say that, being a Brahmin, he had done a wicked act and had fallen from grace. If his offence were sufficiently serious he would become an out-caste and in that event there would be no form of expiation that could restore to him his Brahmin caste.

According to our Brahmin psychiatrist informant, the ordinary caste Hindu sincerely believes that his social condition is due to the working of the moral law of the universe; and that it would be morally wrong and irreligious to seek to interfere with that law by measures for the relief of his condition. This traditional view is based on the Hindu belief in Karma (fate or destiny) – the doctrine that a man reaps as he sows.

The comment needs making here that the views stated above are those of someone who is identified with the system. It may be difficult for a reader who is aware of the size and social complexity of the country concerned to accept them without many reservations, except in so far as they apply to those caste Hindus who are themselves identified with their culture. But it is worth further reflection that the underprivileged classes in Indian society, which must number, perhaps, eighty million people, despite formidable social disabilities and economic hardships, have lived peaceably, on the whole, for centuries, without attempting to raise themselves above the station in life to which they were born. It is evident that the forces maintaining the *status quo* have been very strong and virtually all-pervading in the past, though currently radical changes are taking place in India (see also pp. 86–87).

The introduction of change may be very difficult in a society in which each individual is believed to be responsible for his own spiritual fate. For example, by tradition, the Brahmins are administrators, judges, doctors, and so on; they predominate in every profession. When in war they have to do other things, this can lead to a great deal of conflict if they cannot adjust themselves. So long as they are able to follow occupations that are in conformity with the old traditions their adjustment will not be threatened. In the Brahmin community the head of the family is the dominating figure and the children have no voice. Changed conditions are giving rise to mental conflict and ill-health in that respect. It has been frequently observed that young Brahmins who go abroad often come back disgruntled and cannot settle down; but the older people cannot accept that change is happening in the rest of the world. Such a young Brahmin would not be accepted by his family and would have to live a separate existence elsewhere. The traditionalist view would be that the young Brahmin was delinquent, although the psychiatric view might be that he was maladjusted and, possibly, neurotic.

Nigeria – Society is the Law

According to a Western-trained Nigerian psychiatrist, in Nigeria after the puberty rituals have been completed, society is divested of responsibility, and the child becomes a man and responsible for his own actions. Many Westerners believe that neurosis is rare in primitive societies, but investigations among primitive people in Nigeria show that delinquency and behaviour disorders are well recognized by these peoples and, according to Western psychiatric criteria, come within some category of neurosis. From the point of view of the primitive people, such acts are regarded either as more or less abnormal behaviour or as delinquency, which the group will punish.

Environmental Determinism

A social scientist who has specialized in the study of Soviet Communism suggested that the Soviet version of Marxism has become an ideology comparable with a religious ideology, as a guiding way of life for a large part of the world; that it is more accurate to place Soviet Marxism beside the religions than to consider it *vis-à-vis* democracy.

Reports on the development of psychiatric thought in the U.S.S.R. indicate that there has been some degree of reversal in the interpretation given to individual maladjustment. Earlier it had been a Marxist assumption that social environment was entirely responsible for the behaviour of the individual. This led naturally to the view that defective social institutions were the reason for crime and maladjustment, and that the criminal ought to be treated as if he were ill, because he had grown up in a bourgeois society.

A new situation has now arisen in the Soviet Union with a generation which has grown up for thirty years in a society that is almost by definition considered to be perfect. A new policy is evolving that greatly increases the amount to which the adult is liable to be held responsible for his own deviations and maladjustments. (The deviant individual is now more in the position of a sinner who has been given full understanding of the correct way of life and yet wilfully refuses to behave in that way; subject, of course, to the recognition of diminished responsibility through mental illness.)

The present practice, therefore, is a reversal of the earlier socialist belief that, if the institutions are improved, the individuals will automatically be good, well adjusted, and well functioning. During World War II, there was an instance in the United States of the fallacy of this belief. A newly constructed defence town had been very fully equipped with adequate housing, food, schools, and other services, but no provision was made for services associated with mental illness and family breakdown; so deep was the unacknowledged belief that, if the economic and social conditions were adequately taken care of, there would be no need for such services. Only one psychiatrist was appointed to the staff of the hospital, in order, it was supposed, to deal with cases of mental breakdown due to antecedent conditions; but the load that actually fell upon him and the rest of the hospital staff had been completely unanticipated by the planners.

A Note on Marxist Values in a Confucian Culture

The success of Communism in China has naturally provoked interest in the relationship between Marxism and Confucianism. In both systems man is regarded as not essentially bad and it is believed, in both, that much of the responsibility for ill arises in society. An important difference between them is that Confucianism stresses harmony, the golden mean, adjustment and a harmonious expression of instincts; whereas Soviet Marxism does not. In a Marxist ideal of society, on the contrary, the dominant social class imposes its values on other social classes. The Marxist ideal lies in the field of new states of synthesis arising out of conflicts, not harmony.

IDENTITY

Identity

We have written elsewhere (pp. 1–51) on the subject of identity and, in addition, many of the definitions of mental health touch upon this subject, whenever reference is made to relationships between the individual and the environment. One aspect of identity that is relevant at this stage of our discussion is that of the acceptance of self. Acceptance of the self means acceptance of weakness as well as strength; to do this necessitates the individual becoming free from the harmful effects of emotional con-

Mental Health and Value Systems

flict and also, of anxiety and ignorance. Goethe's *Werde der du bist* (become what you are) points to an important principle. It might be fruitful to find out how the question, 'Who am I?' is answered by people of various religions, and one might anticipate getting many different replies. For example, it might be anticipated that in a Confucian system the answer to this question would be found to lie in the family; whereas in a Hindu society the answer might be affected by acceptance of the principle of reincarnation (see also p. 111).

The way in which this question is answered in different value systems is of considerable importance in international mental health work, and indeed to international relations generally, especially in relation to such issues as human brotherhood and racial equality.

FLEXIBILITY

Hindu Flexibility

A Western-trained Indian psychiatrist has made the observation that it is an important belief of Hinduism, perhaps not widely appreciated, that knowledge of God is continually advancing. There is in Hinduism a general absence of rigid concepts and a flexibility that has permitted members of other religions living in India to follow their faith for centuries; Jews in South India, Parsees after Persia had been overrun, and people of many other religions, too. It is claimed on their behalf that the Indian people have found a certain mental poise and equanimity in the Hindu religion, a poise which they think cannot be acquired through other forms of belief or by material acquisition, wealth, or comfort. The Hindu will accept starvation and poverty because, it is said, he feels that he can adapt himself to his environment and attain mental equanimity and peace.

The flexibility of Hinduism is understandable because, according to our informant, no limitation is set on intellectual beliefs. Hinduism allows absolute liberty of thought and subordinates dogma to experience; which sanctions have enabled the Hindus to vary their notions of God. An illustrative quotation from a Hindu writer reveals a typical Hindu attitude:

'Hinduism is wholly free from the strange obsession of the Semitic faiths that the acceptance of a particular religious metaphysic is necessary for salvation, and non-acceptance thereof is a heinous thing meriting eternal punishment in Heaven.'

Hinduism is flexible in time, in space, and in particular area. In addition there have been many instances in which Hinduism has become modified to meet the impact of other religions, e.g. Buddhism, Christianity, and Islam.

On the other hand, Hinduism controls the social customs, which must be rigidly obeyed by all. Thus the caste system has a synthesis, the broad outline of which can be recognized all over the Indian sub-continent. One effect of this rigidity is that, by accepting limitation of their functions and aspirations, the members of each caste and sub-caste know what is expected of them and do not encroach on the functions of other castes.

Hebrew Flexibility

A Hebrew scholar remarked to us that the flexibility of Judaism becomes apparent when Jewish history and the development of Jewish communities in many countries are considered. The diversity in the interpretation of Judaism is striking; Orthodox (Traditional) Judaism is thousands of years old, but within the past hundred years there have developed the Reform and Liberal movements of Judaism, which differ from Orthodox Judaism in the interpretation of the Jewish faith in many respects.

On deeper study, Jewish thought reveals more flexibility than might appear to those who are unfamiliar with it. It is an important Jewish value that the individual should be able to face up to the problems of the day – not taking refuge in past happenings – essentially to develop the capacity of looking to the future with optimism. This feeling of looking to the future helps to produce flexibility in thinking.

The Moslem Concept of Change

During the course of the discussion on 'values', the Moslem concept of change and relativity in time and space was introduced.

We were informed by a Western-trained Moslem psychiatrist that, in Islam, the concept of relativity has been developed as highly as in any other of the great religions. One of the more influential Islamic philosophies is known as controversialism, also sometimes referred to as the 'fruits of vagueness'. it has been suggested above (p. 89), that the attitude of pious Moslems to the Koran is that it is a book of inspiration rather than an encyclopaedia of conduct. The Prophet said 'My people will never agree in error' – a statement which resulted in the establishment of the doctrine of the Consensus of Opinion. In this doctrine a very high value is set on community responsibility and, in the opinion of our informant, it illustrates not only the high evaluation of the worth of the human mind in Islam, but also that religion is a living institution and not fossilized.

The pious Moslem recognizes that there has been no fresh divine guidance or instruction other than that contained in the scriptures, during the past fourteen centuries, and interprets this to mean that the Creator's intention is that men should use their minds and solve their problems in the light of guidance already given. The Consensus has become one of the major sources of the Islamic Law, and it has had the important result that when a community comes to agree that a certain type of behaviour is antisocial this view will gain legal sanction. With the expansion of the Islamic Commonwealth precedents have been created by analogy.

Since Consensus is unlikely to be secured in regard to attitudes to behaviour deviations, it will follow that, as far as Islamic law is concerned, the concept of mental health and, conversely, mental illness will be vague. The principle is that society does not regard psychiatric problems as coming within the orbit of the religious laws, because the insane (and minors) are not held responsible for their actions. The responsibility of individuals is not held to be modified in cases of mental disorder not amounting to insanity.

It is claimed on behalf of Islam that difficult legal situations do not arise in connection with problems of mental ill-health, because the concept of consensus has enabled the adoption of flexible attitudes to mental illness. This is why in the Sudan, for example, it has not been found difficult to adopt new knowledge into the legal system provided a consensus of opinion can be obtained; and if there is no consensus, precedents are looked for.

We understand that the practical outcome of this situation is that changes in the interest of mental health can be effected easily in an Islamic community provided that the necessary consensus is secured. There is another particular feature of the Islamic world to consider, in that four schools of law exist side by side, based on traditions in different parts of the Islamic Commonwealth at the time they arose. Consequently the solution to difficulties in domestic life and in interpersonal relationships can be sought and generally found in one or other of the four schools. Currently an attempt is being made to unify the four schools and establish a single official Islamic position. Differences between the schools are not basic and the controversies that occur are mainly about non-essentials.

Feeling-tone and Flexibility

An Anglican priest and pastoral psychologist remarked that flexibility is a marked feature of the Anglican position too; and in this case arises out of the dependence upon feeling-tone rather than upon logic. This may be held to apply to English institutions generally, including political life. Perhaps a specific feature of the Anglican attitude is a continuous balance which is maintained between love on the one hand and truth on the other; this balance not infrequently leads to tension. It would probably be true to say that in the ideal it would be held that love should prevail over strict adherence to truth.

Wider Aspects of Flexibility

There are other and wider aspects of flexibility that need to be examined. For example, our informant about Hindu flexibility stated that it is this quality of flexibility in Hinduism that enabled Hinduism 'to meet the impact of other religions'. This would suggest that there are definable limits to the flexibility of Hinduism, limits at which the 'impact' of another religion is 'met'. Continuing our example taken from Hinduism, it has been stated above (pp. 132–3) that Hinduism shows flexibility in time, space, and area. This must be set against some quite definite rigidities; e.g. if a Brahmin contravenes Brahminical rules, he will become an out-caste, and there is no approved way by which such an out-caste can get back his lost status in the same lifetime. Therefore, it would appear that the concept of flexibility in religion needs more exhaustive investigation, which will also take into account family structures and interpersonal relationships within the system.

We are informed that it is possible for four or five religions to be represented within a single Hindu family without causing any very great difficulty; that enough tolerance can be present within a family for the mother to be an orthodox Hindu Brahmin and for a son to be a Christian. Although the mother might regret this situation, as long as the son performs certain little ceremonies no great tensions result. In theory, at least, another son could be a Sikh, another a Buddhist, and a fourth an agnostic.

The above statement will scarcely be acceptable without reservation; but to take it at its explicit value for the purposes of discussion, it needs to be examined in conjunction with the fact to which we have already referred, that, strictly, the contravention of Brahminical rules will result in permanent exclusion from the caste. Thus, in this case, the flexibility shown might not be so much in the conceptual field as in the area of interpretation and application of rules.

The evidence concerning flexibility would appear to be clearer at the level of the community. The presence of flexibility in Hinduism may be illustrated by the fact that there may be members of one Hindu sect which will not kill even an insect, living side by side with another sect which does not object to sacrificing holy animals.

Here again, flexibility at the community level has to be considered in the context of caste rigidity. This will lead us on to further consideration of the question : What is it that is flexible in any religion or ideology? First, in order to clarify our concept of flexibility, let us take an example from the interpretation of scientific hypotheses. A hypothesis will be constructed flexibly in order to take account of various facts as they come to light. Flexibility should not be confused with imprecision of thinking, which is a different order of phenomenon. In religious matters it may happen that an individual does not include precision of thought among his higher personal values and he may be content to live with a relatively undefined belief. His resulting attitude would, no doubt, show an absence of rigidity but this would derive from lack of definition rather than from flexibility.

Flexibility in Period and Geographical Distribution

In regard to period, the relevant question to be considered in relation to any religion or ideology is whether ideas held in the past are still held today, or whether there have been changes in the course of history. In regard to geographical distribution when, for example, considering the Roman Catholic Church as a world-wide body, an impression may be gained of flexibility; Catholicism in France appears to differ in many respects from Catholicism in Canada. Flexibility might also refer to a particular local area; how much flexibility is there within Catholicism in a single area such as, for example, Quebec, at any particular time?

Mental Health and Value Systems

In other words, how much and what kinds of flexibility are allowed within orthodoxy? It may be found that such variations as exist are concerned with practice rather than with principles. The situation can be conceived in which the doctrine may not be flexible but there may be wide variations in interpretation and in the practices arising out of the interpretations. This possibility suggests itself in connection with the Hindu family discussed in the immediately preceding paragraph.

Limits to Flexibility

It was stated by a Roman Catholic theologian that flexibility cannot logically extend to simultaneous acceptance of contradictories. Thus, if one accepts that reason can establish the existence of God, one cannot at the same time say that God does not exist. If one believes that a Revelation was made to man, one cannot at the same time say that possibly no such Revelation was made. If one believes that a Revelation was made (and that its content is true) one then must believe the content of the revelation, and there can be no flexibility on this point. This is often misunderstood as though it meant the arbitrary inventing and laying down of dogmas. A dogma is a proposition explicitly formulated as a statement of truth contained in revelation, and proposed to Catholics to be believed. In such a matter there is nothing to be gained by arguing for flexibility.

Similarly, on the question of behaviour, it is possible by means of the rational analysis of observation, to establish that certain norms exist; and if it is believed that certain modes of action are right, there is no point in arguing flexibility at that point; the question is one of acceptance or rejection.

Flexibility in non-essentials is more open to discussion. There are differences in non-essentials in the Catholic religion, between France and Canada, as indicated in the example taken above; but there is accord on all fundamental propositions of Revelation, on the Hierarchy, and on the moral law. There may be differences of emphasis from place to place. Thus the emphasis in France at the moment on liturgical practice need not necessarily be the case elsewhere.

Toleration of other groups should not be confused with flexibility in doctrine or in norms of behaviour. Thus it is essential, in order to remain a member of the Roman Catholic Church, that one should believe the Church's doctrine. The Church cannot of course compel belief, but a man cannot at the same time remain a member and refuse belief.

Flexibility and Definition

It would be interesting to investigate the proposition that definiteness of conviction may have a considerable influence on the concept of mental health. For example, a comparative study might be made between the concept of mental health held by individuals belonging to a group of young people in a religious organization in which there is a definite common conviction of what is revealed and therefore absolute, and what is not, and of what is true and what is false; in comparison with the concept of mental health held by young people of an organization in which there is a minimum of definite statements about what is true and what is false. This investigation needs to be made in an atmosphere free from any preconception whether it is better or worse, from the point of view of mental health, to have a more, or a less, sharply defined religious attitude.

In discussion the proposition might be advanced that in a group where beliefs are well defined, the mental health of its members may remain at a high level so long as each member accepts the beliefs of the group. But if members have contact with other points of view and if they begin to question things which they have previously regarded as fixed and definite, then mental health difficulties might arise. On the other hand, members of a type of religious organization where beliefs are less closely defined might undergo changes of heart and mind arising from external contacts without a comparable degree of disturbance.

Another aspect of this discussion is the amount of choice

and individual decision that is possessed by members of the group. To belong to a religious organization where beliefs are narrowly defined will leave each member with a range of simple positive or negative choices of acceptance or rejection of positions, as they arise. In a religious group where beliefs are less defined, the members may be faced with making a choice between multiple alternatives. The necessity to make a choice will almost inevitably engender some anxiety in the individual, and it would be legitimate to inquire whether the quality of anxiety in the case of the defined single alternative is different from that inherent in a multiple-choice situation.

The member of the religious organization in which the truth is clear and definite will be exposed to the single but potentially severe anxiety of choosing between belonging and not belonging. His defences against anxiety will need to be constructed against major threats to his position. On the other hand, the member of a religious organization where each member has to make his own analysis and decision of what is true and what is false, on a wide range of alternatives, will need to have defences against constantly recurring anxiety perhaps often of a minor character.

Consequently, if freedom from anxiety were a criterion of mental health (which, though it may have some bearing on the quality of mental health, we would not accept without considerable reservations), it would be possible to argue that it is good to be in a well-defined position, provided that that position is neither shaken nor exposed to disturbing influences. Alternatively, it might be argued that it is good to be in an undefined position in circumstances of rapid change and adaptation. Objective research into this question would be valuable.

SOCIAL ORGANIZATION

In this section certain types of organization will be referred to as illustrations of the kind of factor which the mental health worker must take into consideration in dealing with problems. As in previous sections, the examples quoted are taken from only very few of the widely varying types of organization that can be found. Most of them have been presented through the eyes of someone speaking from within the culture (see also p. 105).

Hindu – the Joint Family System

A Western-trained Indian Brahmin psychiatrist described the Hindu joint family system as a social institution of great importance which, in his opinion, has contributed to the mental health of millions in India. In this system the oldest male is the head of the family and all the members of the family, unmarried sisters, daughters, and grand-daughters of the head of the family, sons and their wives, grandsons and their wives – in fact, several generations – reside in the family house; and each person has a right to be fed and clothed by the head of the family, from the common property. This system, we are told, promoted family solidarity and helped to provide support for the aged and infirm, the orphans and the poor relatives. Traditionally, India has not had a poor-law system or indigenous institutions to care for the sick.

As the younger members of the family have no need to seek work, they are not exposed to work anxiety. In such a system the senior woman wields great authority in domestic matters, and it is her duty to see that the children get as much attention as they need. The system is also conducive to early marriage and child marriages, as the young males are not expected to support their wives; but, among its disadvantages, the Hindu joint family system tends to discourage initiative and to stifle enterprise.

Owing to conditions of modern life the system is breaking up, which many people in India believe to be a major cause of psycho-neurosis, because when members become deprived of family solidarity they have neither financial stability nor other forms of security. Youths will find that, unless they are able to earn enough to support their wives, they cannot hope to get married.

According to the views expressed to us, there are three important factors in the Hindu religion in respect of family life. One is to make children indispensable and to foster the desirability of every family having children. This is effected by making the male child, in particular, essential in the performance of certain ceremonies which help to keep the ancestors safe in heaven. These religious demands ensure not only that every family has children but that the male children are looked after with great care and receive maternal and paternal love.

The second factor is the principle that women should stay at home and not go out to work. Most of Hindu teaching on the family is aimed to keep the women at home and to ensure that the children receive all their mother's attention. Today, however, more and more women leave their homes, in addition to the out-caste women who have traditionally supplied much of the available labour force. We are told that this has led to the neglect of children.

The third factor is that of early marriage, together with the selection of the bride by the parents of the bridegroom. This, the people believe, helps to eliminate mental illness and neurosis (in so far as the latter is recognized) because the selection is made only from certain families whose genealogy is well known to the people concerned. If the descent has been in any way consanguineous, the marriage will not be contracted, because of the prevalent fear of the inheritability of mental illness and neurosis. Another check is made through the horoscopes which are prepared at the birth of each child. After consultation with the parents of the possible brides and after studying the various horoscopes, the parents of the bridegroom will decide which of the families among the selection are likely to perpetuate trouble and which are not.

The Hindu religion also provides that when there are no children in the family, a boy must be adopted from another family. The adoption is necessary because of the son's duty to perform the ancestor veneration ceremonies to which we have referred above. There is another objective, in that a system of adoption helps to ensure that all male children are looked after by a mother and that she gives them her tenderness, care, and affection.

Another feature of Hindu family life, according to our informant, is that, as far as possible, the father is kept with the family. That has been achieved by the rigid caste system in India. Through the centuries, in times of war, the man with a trade has not been called up. Only the fighter has gone to war. His family has known that and has been duly prepared, and has therefore not suffered from last-minute conflicts about his leaving. Each man, by sticking to his province, has been able to maintain his family as far as possible without disintegration.

A modern difficulty (as seen by the caste member) has been that with the tendency of the system to disintegrate, opposition from out-castes has greatly multiplied. A great deal of the conflict has followed the return of untouchables after receipt of a Western education.

Confucianism – Social Role

A Chinese specialist in comparative education expressed the the view that one of the contributions of Confucianism to mental health has related to definiteness in role-determination. A father knows clearly how he should act towards his son, and the son toward his father; the roles of brother, wife, mother or friend, are equally definitely determined. This helps to remove uncertainty, fear, and insecurity from interpersonal relations and, in the opinion of many people who are identified with the culture, facilitates the development and maintenance of mental health.

The question may be posed : where the mother is uncertain about how to love her child and, in particular the proper way in which to express her love, are there more or fewer problems of adjustment than in the case of the traditional Chinese attitude where the mother knows clearly and definitely how she should go about it? It seems possible that mothers in Western society are less certain how to express their love for their children. The effects of definiteness of roles, especially those relating to mother and child interaction, need to be explored.

One striking characteristic of the Confucian system is that it gives concrete descriptions of what is meant by 'good'. The possible inference from our previous discussion that a clear delineation of roles is conducive to mental health, except in societies which are rapidly changing, is interesting in view of the comparatively high degree of resistance that Confucianism has shown to cultural change. In the Confucian description, the roles of parents are restricted to a range of human behaviour which is constant whatever changes society may undergo.

> Confucian teaching, we are told, is that however old a man may be, he cannot be happy unless he is in harmony with his father. This does not mean that a man is required to obey his father blindly. A man will be in harmony with his father when he fulfils the role of an ideal son, and the father the role of an ideal father. It is important to note that the Confucian delineation of role is largely the defining of social relationships with respect to the person taking the role. Ideal social relationships are laid down as the norm to be followed.

We would note that the use of the term 'role', however fashionable it may be at present in social science circles, is likely to raise difficulties of individual interpretation. Some of these difficulties will relate to the degree of personal identification with an affective investment in the role that the term will imply.

The Jewish Family

> A Hebrew scholar has pointed out that the Bible shows the place of family love and affection in the history of the Jewish people. In Judaism, the baby is regarded as coming from God and is welcomed with great love from the moment of birth. Girls are not less welcome than boys. The history of persecution has indicated the strength of Jewish family life in periods of great stress.
>
> Hebrew wisdom stresses that the home is the training-

ground for the individual; and that the value of holiness is more than an abstraction. There are many Jewish people who, although they may not be devout, like the feeling of warmth from religion mainly for social reasons. The Jewish home, according to our informant, has to be integrated into the general pattern of social progress and to be made the training-ground for the individual. The parents are regarded as educators. Long before the child goes to school it is the responsibility of parents to introduce certain duties to the child.

The authority of parents does not derive from the fact that they are older or stronger, or that they are the originators of their children's lives. Their physical and other advantages over their children impose on them essential responsibilities, especially to educate and inspire their children with an appreciation of the holiness of life. The vital point is made in Rabbinic teaching that if a father should order his children to commit an offence, however slight, against other human beings, he should not be obeyed.

Islam – Filial Piety

We understand that in Islam the community and the family are the two corner-stones of human relations. The family is brought up in filial piety and in the appreciation of the authority of the father over his household. These relations are almost of a religious character, but as has been already discussed, Islam has made allowances for the biological need of human beings for change, in the long run. The Prophet's son-in-law, Ali, said, 'People may resemble their times more closely than their parents.'

The Nigerian Family

We are informed that, in most of the Nigerian tribes, the father is the head of the home, dictates the customs of the family, and governs the behaviour of the child. A child in Africa knows what to do in most circumstances. Most of the customs represent ideals that have been laid down as a traditional system of behaviour. However, traditional behaviour is by no means rigid and through the years the principles governing behaviour have been in a state of continuous change. Even at periods when the outside influences appear to have been inconsiderable there has been a steady process of modification of attitude, which has resulted in the customs of the people being subjected to change.

Differing Patterns in Family Life

In studying the important question of the interrelationship between family patterns of living and the concepts of mental health in various religions and ideologies, attention should be directed to the study of what happens in society and families when the new generation takes over from its predecessors.

Among different societies a wide variety of patterns can be seen during the process of handing on authority from one generation to the next. Distinctions have been drawn, for example, between parent-oriented 'vertical', and sibling-oriented 'horizontal', societies.

There was discussion of an apparent paradox in Confucian society between its rigid organization, on the one hand, and its dependence upon induced moral principles, with a denial of revelation, on the other. It was suggested that it would be reasonable to suppose that a sibling-oriented society might be favourable to an empirical approach to morality; whereas a parent-oriented society might be conducive to revelation and authority. Whatever this apparent paradox may be due to, and it is a vast subject for study, it might be said that in Confucian society the question of handing power from one generation to another has been given a narrowly defined institutional form.

Other societies have adopted other ways. Generally speaking in a sibling-oriented society, sibling organization results in the displacement, to a greater or lesser degree, of the parent-figure. When this happens social institutions come into being to deal with sibling rivalry. Further, it is important to consider what is the fate of the father figure in a sibling-oriented society. This is a wide question which deserves a great deal more study. Some hypothetical questions can be asked. For example, if the father had been the dominant leader of the horde, when the siblings had dealt with the situation was the father-figure left in subjection? It might be felt that this is the situation in societies where an authoritarian régime has been violently overthrown by a popular revolution. If the deposed father-figure is still feared, he and the system he has represented may be strongly repressed, regarded with hate as traitorous, and this hatred will be reflected in the attitudes of the new régime. Or he may have been left as a loved father-figure, shorn of responsibility but retaining the authority inherent in a positive relationship. Such a situation may lead to compromise and a more continuous process of handing over power. In addition to the residual attitude to the deposed father-figure, the course of subsequent history may depend also upon the effectiveness of the institutions devised to control the effects of sibling rivalry.

This field of study is virtually unexplored, from the point of view of the sciences of human behaviour, but it would appear to have great relevance to the proper understanding of historical events.

CONCEPTS OF RIGHT AND WRONG

The Group and the Individual

Among the emphases, which differ in various cultures, that are laid on aspects of child upbringing, those which are given to the introduction of concepts of right and wrong to the child will show wide variations. Among the important points to consider are, at what stage of development is the child brought face to face with the difference between right and wrong, and by whom? (See also pp. 96–97.)

It appears to many people brought up in a Western culture that the relationship with a particular adult, parent or teacher, becomes important for the definition of right and wrong very early in the child's life. The withdrawal of love or the giving of punishment creates an attitude towards right and wrong in which the first notion of guilt may develop.

A distinction is sometimes made between guilt and shame, in respect of the attitude of society to right and wrong. Thus a so-called 'guilt' culture is one in which the individual's own identifications are largely responsible for determining his conduct; whereas a 'shame' culture is one in which conduct is determined by the invocation of the approval, or more particularly the disapproval, of the group attitudes in which the individual concerned will concur.

In *Islam,* as discussed on pages 119–120, concepts of good and evil and of mental health are very complex and continually changing. Something of what is regarded today as 'mental health', the earlier Moslem teachers would, on the whole, have regarded in terms of an interaction between evil and good. There are people, belonging to many religions, who believe that good itself can never reach the ultimate goal unless it interacts with evil. In earlier times moral and religious teachings and injunctions in Islam were largely in relation to personal, family, and group ethics and, it is presumed, would have appeared to the people of the time as adequate for the needs and welfare of society.

In many religions and not only in Islam, notions of good and evil – and mental health and ill-health with which they may sometimes be identified – are relative to time and space; and, as we have discussed on page 120, something which is regarded as compatible with mental health today might be regarded as harmful tomorrow. Moslem religious thinkers, however, have been particularly aware of the effects of change on the needs of their societies. Our Islamic informant emphasized that the 'ecological' concept in religion (as this attitude might be termed) has been the basis and the major cause of the proliferation of sects, tenets, and schools which has characterized Islam, especially during the medieval period. This, of course, was a period when geographical and

148

cultural differences between the countries of the Islamic world were all the more marked because of the difficulty of communication.

Aspirations and Mental Health

It has been stated that mental health demands good interpersonal relations and this statement, in relation to a given society, can be either a description or an aspiration. At a descriptive level the example could be taken of a very simple society which was carrying on an undisturbed tradition of cannibalism. If in such a society the notion had never been introduced that cannibalism was wrong (perhaps as a result of lack of exposure to the values of other societies), it could be said that cannibals could enjoy good mental health, provided that they followed the rules and conventions of their society about whom to eat and in what circumstances, and that these conditions were clearly defined. However, if it should happen that a large majority of the members of this primitive society were to adopt, as an aspiration, the notion that good interpersonal relations could not include cannibalism, then it could no longer be said that the cannibals among them were mentally healthy. In other words, if mental health is invoked in an aspirational rather than a descriptive sense the situation alters at once.

In this whole discussion we are taking mental health more from the point of view of an aspiration, and our interest is in whether a certain order of aspiration in mental health, whatever it may be, is admissible to a society. Mental health as an aspiration should not be confused with an aspiration in relation to goodness and truth.

The effects of such confusion can be illustrated by an example from India.

It has been stated to us by a Brahmin that, in the estimation of Indian caste society, the acceptance of their inferior position by untouchables does not reflect upon their state of mental health. On the other hand, an outsider, using the term 'mental health' in an aspirational sense to include some concept of human equality, would not agree that the acceptance of an inferior position was compatible with good mental health.

However, this is not a true antithesis, because two separable factors are being considered together. In a society in which equality is not a possible aspiration, from a descriptive point of view the mental health of the untouchable may be good; but where mental health as an aspiration is possible, a high level of mental health would be incompatible with acceptance of outcaste status.

In Asia generally, today, change is occurring in most countries, in that a greater emphasis is being laid on stated goals for human endeavour. In other words, more and more, mental health is approaching an aspirational level. In India there has been a marked modification of the traditional position in regard to concepts of caste and out-caste in society.

Mental health (and also social change from an aspirational point of view) is not at all the same thing as a search for the good and the beautiful; which can occur in a society in which social change is not a possible aspiration. In the past it has not been uncommon for aspirations towards abstract ideals to be included as part of a written constitution that allowed for no social change; though the modern trend is for aspirations towards social change also to be included in the constitutions of newly emerging states.

Attitudes to Sexuality

We understand that the recognition of sexuality is an integral part of the Confucian definition of a human being, and is to be given due harmony of expression. As far as the Chinese Confucian attitude is concerned, there appears to be some difference between precept and practice. Though sexuality may be defined as being part of life, it appears that people tend to look forward to the second half of adult life when the trials and turbulence of family life will have been passed, and when sexuality will no longer be an important issue for the individual.

Relevant Material from Various Religions and Ideologies

Chinese attitudes to sexuality need to be considered also in relation to the style of interpersonal relationships that exist in the society, about which comparatively little is known from a psychological point of view. It might be argued that sexuality in a Confucian society is stressed mainly as an integral part of the parental role, an attribute of the child as a prospective parent and of the adult during the reproductive period, but not of the adult in later life.

Among Christians, likewise, the observer may become aware of differences between precept and practice. It would be generally true of Christians that sexuality is regarded as a natural function of the individual, that is, a personal attribute that will subserve interpersonal relationships. As might be expected, many differences will be found among the attitudes of individuals and groups. The Roman Catholic view is that sexuality, because it is a natural function, is intrinsically good, but can be misused. In the Calvinist view, there has been more emphasis, on the one hand, on the evil and corruption of the unregenerate flesh and, on the other hand, on the potentiality of regeneration, on salvation and becoming perfect through Grace. The degree to which sexual behaviour is controlled and regulated strictly by means of social institutions that, in the case of nearly all Christians, acquire some sacramental value, suggests that very strong psychological forces are operating. Another indication of the strength of the forces involved is the degree to which guilt tends to become attached to sexuality, particularly to sexual behaviour that is not protected by the sanction of a religious institution; and this might be regarded as characteristic of the Christian attitude. Thus it has come about that the Christian teaching on sexuality has sometimes been mistaken to mean that all sexuality is sin, and that salvation depends on the total repudiation of sexuality. There have been instances in history in which a whole community has taken this view.

Again, attitudes to sexuality need further examination in the light of the style of interpersonal relationships that prevails in family life among Christians. On the whole, the kind of intimate emotional relationships that are fostered in the monogamous Christian family may be of a rather different order from those of the joint family in which there may be more than one wife and in which women generally occupy a position of marked inferiority. In the monogamous family, emotional intensity will tend to be higher; and guilt, when it occurs, may be intense also. In respect of Christians among whom sexuality is an individual attribute which subserves interpersonal relationships, the individual's problems of sexuality are less likely to be resolved by the passage of time in the way that appears to be a feature of attitudes to sexuality among Chinese families.

In Hindu India, we are told, there is a general tendency to view sexuality not primarily in terms of procreation; at least equally important will be the pleasure involved. There are, however, important exceptions to this among Indian communities, a striking example being found among the Jains, who reject the erotic values of sexuality to almost an extreme degree.

Islamic teaching has a great deal to say about the family but our informant states that, in the Koran, the biological function of sex is valued for reasons of population and the emphasis is on procreation.

Attitudes to Error: Marxism in Confucian Society

It appears to some members of the Committee that a difference between Confucianism and Soviet Communism can be seen in the attitudes that have been reported of Chinese Communists towards the individual who does not admit the truth as the others see it. The Russian attitude, we understand, has tended to be that the best solution to such a problem is to liquidate the aberrant individual, on the grounds that people who have been brought up under a bourgeois régime are probably irredeemable. This attitude has been expressed particularly strongly against people who have appeared at one time to conform, and then have deviated from acceptable doctrine.

Relevant Material from Various Religions and Ideologies

It has been reported, in respect of the revolution in China, that there is a considerable contrast in the approach of Chinese Communists to those who, in a comparable phase of the Soviet revolution, would have been regarded as irreclaimable. The Chinese Communists are reported to have kept much of the traditional Soviet practice of a pressured confession, but to place more emphasis upon the innate goodness of the individual which makes it possible for him, after confession and conversion, to be redeemed rather than liquidated. The practices associated with these efforts at conversion are popularly called 'brainwashing', but it is said that perhaps 'mind purification' would be a more correct analogy.

The term, 'brainwashing' has come to be used, in the West, in the sense of obliterating an individual's highest values, and it has also been used, with unfortunate connotations, by those who are hostile to psychotherapeutic practice.

The use of a more precise term might have enabled a truer understanding of what is involved to have permeated the West. Proper international understanding demands the avoidance of action that may increase prejudice, such as the bandying about of names or expressions that themselves adversely affect understanding. Our example has drawn attention to the fact that a negative attitude drawn from political strife can, in certain circumstances, become attached to psychotherapeutic endeavour, and this is of such importance that we should like to consider it further.

False Analogies of the Therapeutic Process

It appears to us that there is a great danger to the whole of mental health endeavour in some of the analogies that have been drawn between, and identifications made, of therapeutic psychiatric practice with other processes that have resulted in an individual's change of attitude. 'Brainwashing' has been cited above as an example of the hostile misuse of a concept, in the form of a damaging analogy. There are others that might be quoted; for example, catharsis, in the sense used in

Greek tragedy; and the experiences leading up to religious conversion.

These processes have in common the notion of purification – the getting rid of evil from the system, cleansing, and renewal – which will be applicable also to some aspects of psychotherapy, especially in respect of such processes as abreaction, interpretation, and transference identification. The danger of such an analogy to mental health practice is that the attitude to the analogical process may be projected on to psychotherapy.

To the classical Greek, the catharsis in tragedy was both cleansing and ennobling, an experience that strengthened identification with the values of society. The same is true, today, of what society regards as 'great' art, in all its forms, at least to those who are identified with the value system. To outsiders who have neither sympathy nor empathy with the system, such catharsis may appear in a very different light – as obscurantism or as a binding of the individual still more firmly in the chains of his delusion.

In relation to the processes of religious conversion such antitheses of attitude can be even more striking. To the co-religionist, conversion will be a matter of rejoicing, a victory and an increase in identity strength. To those whom the converted person has left, conversion will be a matter of defeat, of loss of identity strength, of sorrow, resentment, and, perhaps, retaliation.

In the case of political conversion, as we have seen, one and the same process is capable of appearing to opponents as the washing away of the person's highest values and as a corruption; and to the protagonists as a reclamation and as a fulfilment.

It appears to us that mental health practitioners should take careful note of the difficulties and dangers of such attitude projections. Inasmuch as psychotherapy usually involves the changing of patients' attitudes, it is important that the psychotherapeutic agencies should be acceptable to the community, because if it should happen that psychotherapy should be regarded by the society as something alien or antipathetic, the danger will arise of attracting the kind of negative attitude evident in the 'brainwashing' name-calling cited above. We shall be referring later (pp. 183–7) to some of the difficulties which may be experienced during the treatment of psychotics, when an attempt is made by means of psychotherapy and other forms of treatment to get psychotic people to change their attitudes.

The Moslem Concept of Utility

It has often been pointed out that the theory or principle of Islamic teaching is that it is egalitarian, it does not recognize classes and castes, and regards all human beings as equal. However, it appears that practice varies widely from precept in this respect in Islamic, as in other societies, and the Moslem concept of utility, to which we have already referred on page 120, is of interest here. For example, at first sight it might be held that polygamy rests on the antithesis of an egalitarian principle but, we are informed, the justification of polygamy in the minds of Moslems is biological and not moral. Thus, although Islam has sanctioned polygamy, it has also created impediments to it. The Prophet laid down the principle of the absolute equality of the wives and also maintained that polygamy was the worst practice permitted to Moslems.

A modern attitude to polygamy was expressed by a Moslem psychiatrist who had been trained in the West. He emphasized that polygamy was sanctioned because of its important survival value, the conclusion having been drawn from historical evidence that at many times in history whole communities, especially those nomadic societies where manpower is of major importance in survival, would have died out but for polygamy. It is further believed that in such nomadic societies there is hardly any evidence that polygamy has an adverse effect on the mental health of women in polygamous households, and, in particular, that jealousy is not manifest.

Mental Health and Value Systems

The comment might be added here that, as in the cases of attitudes to the practices of female circumcision and routine tonsillectomy (see pp. 89–90), more evidence of disturbance arising out of polygamy might have been found had it been possible to conduct the search with modern insights into human relations, and had the women concerned been in a position to conceptualize another form of family relationships. The very complacency of the women under such conditions would need to be appraised, along with their other attitudes.

It has been reported of the Sudan, and no doubt of other places in the Islamic world as well, that polygamous families are tending to break down and that the attitude of the community to the practice is undergoing change. We have been informed that with the progressive urbanization of the society and the increasing availability of efficient health services, a reduction in child mortality and a significant raising of the expectations of life are changing the whole population balance. In some areas, instead of the age-long numerical deficiency of men, the reverse has happened, e.g. in Khartoum alone there are stated to be some ten thousand fewer women than men. In such circumstances the practice of polygamy comes to be recognized as detrimental to the welfare of society, a change of attitude that is strongly reinforced when the women in the society become aware of other forms of family life that exist in other countries.

This is an illustration of a human institution which, for centuries, has been valued as a 'good' and justified on 'ecological' grounds; but which has now gradually come to be recognized by many people as 'bad'. We are informed that this situation is being interpreted in the Sudan as being mainly a public health problem and a matter neither for legislation nor for moral sanctions. It has been concluded there that all that was necessary to combat polygamy, once it was recognized as 'bad' by the leaders, was the development of effective maternal and child welfare centres, better health services for the community in general, a reduction in

156

infantile mortality, and an increase in the expectation of life. This has been freely interpreted in the Sudan, we understand, as an example of how scientific measures have helped to avoid severe social friction which would have been based partly on religious feelings.

It may not be universally agreed that the utilitarian explanation of these changing phenomena completely covers the case, and it may be felt that the element of better information, of greater knowledge of the outside world, may at least have accelerated the change of attitude. There may be other important factors, too. Since it is the case today that, even in relatively underdeveloped countries, more and more women are making wider and wider personal contacts, through increasing industrialization and working in the factories and travel outside the narrow confines of the village, it is relevant to inquire what will be the effects on the traditional Moslem family as an institution, as women by working in the factories tend to become more independent of male authority in the home?

The answer, according to our Moslem informant, is that any change that fulfils the doctrine of utility and which does not run seriously counter to basic religious beliefs, would probably be acceptable in the long run, but this could not be stated with certainty (see also p. 120).

DIFFERENT ATTITUDES TO
SUFFERING – DEATH – GUILT

Christian attitude of Positive Acceptance
According to a pastoral psychologist, the Anglican accepts pain and suffering as a necessary part of life, as if it were a growing edge at which there is continuous endeavour to bring good out of evil and to extract order from disorder, but without any suggestion that evil is anything but evil. Anglicanism has no clear-cut doctrine on this point; such indeed would not be typical of English attitudes. But its

teaching here represents the convergence of two attitudes; the predominance-seeking 'success' attitude which Christianity inherited from Judaism; tempered by the opposite attitude of withdrawal, characteristic of a more Oriental quest for personal salvation. The strong reaction that took place during the sixteenth century ('the Reformation') was in many respects a return to the ethics of Judaism, and caused a rift in Christendom which has yet to be resolved. In its constant attempt to find 'the mean between two extremes' (the phrase is taken from the Introduction to the Book of Common Prayer) Anglicanism finds its *raison d'être*. It believes that this attitude of 'positive acceptance' of suffering approximates to the intentions of Christ. The symbolism of Cross and Resurrection is not to be understood in the sense of being 'saved from' adversity – a misinterpretation that has been responsible for much neuroticism in religion – but as being 'saved through' adversity, the discovery in the experience itself of a deeper level of life, which is to be regarded not as incorporation into the divine so much as the admission of the divine into the human.

The injunction to 'love thy neighbour as thyself' implies the acceptance of one's neighbour. An attitude of mind in which 'success' is a high value will tend to depreciate one's neighbour; an attitude of withdrawal to depreciate the self. The attitude of Christ, particularly in the Sermon on the Mount, is in this sense unique, that it seeks to combine these attitudes (so escaping the dilemma which they usually present) and to create a new completeness of human nature. But guilt and self-hatred, which are endemic in human experience, are not so easily exorcized. Disease, for instance, is often accepted as a substitute for the suffering which real acceptance of life would entail. In practice, therefore, Anglicanism tends to be a Christian version of Stoicism, and to that extent to fall short of its ultimate intention.

A Roman Catholic psychologist pointed out that the Church's attitude to suffering and death was a positive one. The doctrine of the Resurrection, which for St. Paul was the keystone of the faith, meant victory over death. This does not mean that the believing Catholic has no fear of death. He has a natural fear of dying, but can still die happily in the knowledge of an after-life and resurrection. The attitude to suffering likewise is a positive one. The Christian is one who 'takes up the cross daily', so much so that without the cross, we are unworthy of being called 'disciple'. This does not mean that the Christian makes no effort to relieve suffering. He tries, through the love of his neighbour supernaturalized in the love of God, to relieve as much unnecessary suffering as he can. He does not think of suffering as being in itself a good thing, but rather as being (*a*) to some extent unavoidable in this life, and (*b*) capable of being used, by voluntary cheerful acceptance, for the perfecting of man, on both the natural and the supernatural planes.

Confucian Attitude, Suffering not a Positive Value

Confucians, we are told, make no mention in sacred writings of the moral value of suffering as such, but some reference is made to the educational value of adversity in early life. It is doubtful if Confucians would give suffering the positive value of something they actively sought.

A Western-trained Chinese psychiatrist, in discussing the problem of guilt in relation to suffering, has pointed out that in Confucian China the distinction between guilt and shame might not be as clear as has sometimes been suggested. In Chinese culture there is a great deal of inner personal feeling of righteousness which has to do with how one looks to other people. The conscious experiencing of guilt might be different, and if a child learns guilt via shame, it might well be a different experience when it emerges. The distinction is important and might make a difference in the handling of people.

Suffering – the 'Tragedy of Life'

It is a commonly held opinion among medical people that all unnecessary suffering ought to be removed. We would like to inquire whether any broad systems of belief are known of where suffering is considered to be a good thing?

It has been stated above that for the Sikh martyrdom is good, but martyrdom cannot be equated with suffering. The Sikhs set a high value on the strength of the individual to rise above circumstances.

A Western psychiatrist, speaking of the desirability of removing unnecessary suffering, added that, 'It is neither possible nor desirable to abolish the tragedy of life' (see p. 92). This remark deserves further examination. First, it would be highly doubtful whether anybody has ever set out to abolish the tragedy of life with any belief that it might be possible to do so. Secondly, the concept of life free from suffering would be a different order of concept from that which humanity recognizes as life. It might be held that the quality of happiness experienced by an individual would bear some relation to the quality of suffering experienced by him also. In the world of reality there is a great deal of suffering and it might be contended that some of it is unnecessary, in the sense that there is probably a threshold above which suffering will tend to destroy happiness rather than supply any quality to it; and also in the sense that above the threshold no biological nor moral purpose can be seen.

The arguments that have been employed against the use of analgesia in childbirth have usually been based on a feeling that suffering in childbirth is a necessary ingredient for the full development of mother love; a proposition that has found no support in objective observation.

It will probably be widely agreed in most cultures that for the production of the complete human being some element of tragedy in life is essential, but in using the word 'tragedy' it should not be implied that the pattern of tragedy is completed, as in a play. In life no tragedy will be complete until death has occurred, if indeed it is complete then. If the word tragedy in this sense is combined with some concept of hope remaining, the meaning will be clearer.

Relevant Material from Various Religions and Ideologies

A Western-trained Brahmin psychiatrist drew our attention to the existence of one community in India in which it is believed that the major purpose for which children are born is to suffer. As soon as a child is born the community joins together in weeping and wailing; and with equal logic, death is greeted with rejoicing in the community. These people will refuse anaesthetics for surgical operations. They accept completely that life is tragic.

Death – a Hindu View

Our Brahmin informant remarked that, according to Hindu belief, death is a deliverance from suffering in this world; that Hindus are tired of life and desire to go to a happier world; that in principle they welcome death and have no fear. This, it has been said, is one of the reasons why medical progress has been so slow in India, as long as it has been widely considered impious to interfere with the natural course of illness with a view to prolonging life.

Before the above view can be accepted wholly, it is necessary to consider the degree of identification of the individual with the culture belief. Thus, undoubtedly, very many individual Hindus both fear death and are anxious to secure medical treatment for their ailments. But it may be a true generalization that there is a greater tendency towards apathetic acceptance of death and suffering among Hindus than is typical of most other religions.

Suffering and Death – the Sikh View

An anthropologist who has studied the Sikh religion has concluded that the Sikh religion does not hold that death is a value. Death is accepted on a level with a number of other things. It is not taken apart as a particular kind of traumatic experience. To say that there is a fear of death rather than a fear of other kinds of deprivation is to mistake the situation. The Sikh does not think that he is reincarnated necessarily in a human being; but the concept of the 'Ideal Sikh' is so valuable to him that death may represent a lesser deprivation than deformity.

Mental Health and Value Systems

Death – a Nigerian Attitude

Among Nigerian tribes the question of pain is dealt with in a traditional way by the people, especially in connection with death. Where it is recognized that death is painful there are cultural safety-valves made for children. They are allowed to see death in a cultural way, in the sense that the dead person will be coming back. Children just born are often given the name of a person who has just died. Therefore death tends not to be identified with pain, as such.

ATTITUDES TOWARDS MENTAL ILLNESS

Cultural and Religious Influences

At first sight, at least in some countries, public attitudes towards mental illness may appear to be more clearly defined than the corresponding attitudes towards mental health, but, in fact, this is a field about which there is practically no reliable, scientifically based information. Apparently, the specific positions that people take up towards mental abnormality are determined very largely by cultural and religious attitudes, for example, mental illness has frequently been conceived as a form of possession.

To take an illustration from Islam, where the concept of demoniacal possession is usually quite specific; in the Sudan, we are informed by a psychiatrist, illness is regarded as retribution from God, the evil spirit being sent to occupy the individual as a punishment. Thus there is there a concept of sin related to mental illness, and it is contended that illness is due to conflict in the human being between the forces of evil and the forces of virtue. Naturally, and particularly in more primitive communities, such attitudes will be accompanied by primitive treatment methods : i.e. flagellation, starvation, and sequestration from the community, all of which will aim at expulsion of the demon. There is often the additional feeling that mental illness signifies that the individual is not fitted to his community; but it does not always

162

follow that not to be adapted is considered the same as mental illness.

In Western Europe and North America, where there is a certain pride taken in a more sophisticated attitude towards these matters, the ordinary person is not much more than one generation removed from the kinds of attitude which result from belief in the demoniacal origin of mental illness. Even today, examples of these attitudes can be seen not far removed from the surface. On the other hand, in Western psychiatry it can be seen that psychiatric symptoms throughout history have been interpreted in various frames of reference, which have been constantly in change. Thus the frames of reference by which mental illness has been interpreted have included at least four main kinds, and emphases in time have been roughly in the following order:

1. *Transcendental – metaphysical:* God, the Cosmos, the Devil.

2. *Experiential:* life events and happenings to the individual.

3. *Social:* deleterious economic factors and social conditions of living.

4. *Psychobiological:* genetic influences, developmental disorders, damage, and disease.

Among examples of the first group, there are societies which have an angelic theory of mental illness, believing that the persons affected have been touched by the supernatural and chosen for the purposes of God. While both treatment and outcome might be different where an angelic rather than a demoniac theory is held, a psychiatrist might find that the mechanisms in the two cases are very similar. Some people who are regarded by their society as mystics are typical examples of what psychiatrists would regard as sufferers from mental disorder. In the Sudan, often they are endowed with oracular powers by popular imagination and are highly respected and feared.

The Irish name for a mental defective means 'a person who belongs especially to God'.

The above represent a few examples of notions about illness that are current today. As mental health work spreads into new areas it will be very important to investigate these and other attitudes.

SIMILARITIES

Parallels among the Great Religions

In Chapter 2 we have been concerned with variations and differences between the great religions and ideologies. The existence also of similarities must not be overlooked, but this vast field is too great to include in the present study. However, it will be advantageous here to give a brief illustration of some existing tendencies of religions and ideologies to coincide in essentials. For instance, the four groups of Yoga have some equivalents in Christianity, and it is possible, even probable, that parallels may be drawn from other religions too.

There are a number of ancient Sanskrit writings on mental health, on how to attain it, and how to avoid mental illness, etc. It has been represented to us that the word 'Yoga' has been abused in translation; essentially it means communion or rapport with God or the Supreme Being, a state that, in classical literature, has widely been regarded as the optimum condition of mankind. There are four ways in which it is said that such rapport can be obtained. The first is Jnana Yoga, which brings perfect health by the pursuit of intellectual studies – study in order to achieve union with God, which has as its parallel the *intelligo ut credam* of St. Augustine. The second is Hata Yoga, which brings perfect peace and equanimity through the renunciation of the things of the flesh – this will correspond with the mortified Christian life and also with the Judaic conception of submission to the Law and the repression of undesirable or immoral life. The third is Dhama Yoga, which brings health through devotion and which advocates peace through prayer in the temples – this may correspond to St. Anselm's *credo ut intelligam*, devotion in order to understand the mysteries. The fourth is Karma Yoga, which brings health through action; those who work fall into this last group, it is their duty which brings them the peace of mind they seek. This corresponds closely with both the Christian and the Judaic concept of the place of the daily occupation in the religious life.

If the analogies are pursued into Islam the same situation may apply. With the exception of the fourth, they also appear to apply to the Confucian way of life. We might also inquire whether, in Confucianism, the place of daily labour in ordinary life is highly valued.

Setting aside for the moment such bimodalities of terminology as: will and passion, intellect and sense, and thought and action, it might be generally accepted as a proposition that the human being functions at both affective and cognitive levels. Affect and cognition may coincide or they may be in conflict. If they coincide, then the affective help given to the cognitive movement is valuable, if the latter is itself valuable. If they are in conflict, the point of interest to our study is whether, in the society concerned, life will be ruled by emotional or by rational factors. The hope is that the factors would coincide.

It might be possible to get agreement on the proposition that if the cognitive life is helped by and not blocked by affective factors and if the affective factors do not rule life, mental health will be promoted. This principle might be applicable in all of the great religions.

SUMMARY

Among the many variations that occur between different religions and ideologies, a number of contrasting tendencies in human behaviour can be identified. These appear in various combinations in different societies. Some examples are discussed. In much of the world value systems appear to be regarded as fixed but in some cases change and development are allowed for (the Islamic principle of utility is an example).

Mental Health and Value Systems

Man is regarded as perfectible. Among others, this is an important Confucian principle; and values are described in terms of social roles and behaviour, harmony and the Golden Mean. Hinduism places less emphasis on the moral significance of social behaviour, and also regards some kinds of social deviation as a mark of sanctity.

Many religions have emphasized the non-material aspects of their value systems which, in the case of the revealed religions, are of a transcendental order.

Attitudes to human responsibility have, at one extreme, Man as naturally good and wrong development as due to the environment; and at the other extreme, Man as capable of choosing evil even in perfect social conditions. Confucians hold society responsible for wrong behaviour, but the individual is obliged to cultivate the good that is within him. The Hindu projects responsibility into future reincarnations. Many societies, including the Nigerian, divest the society of responsibility for the individual; and this is apparently becoming true also of second-generation Soviet Marxism.

Practically all religions claim some degree of flexibility, but concepts vary. Hinduism allows absolute liberty of thought and subordinates dogma to experience, but controls social behaviour to an uncommon degree. The Hebrew religion gives the impression of rigidity, but has proved remarkably flexible in its application through the centuries.

Flexibility can be institutionalized, as in the Moslem philosophy of controversialism, the 'fruits of vagueness', and the principle of consensus. Consensus, based on feeling-tone, gives flexibility to Anglican Christianity.

The revealed religions tend to be flexible both in period and in geographical distribution, but there is a limit to flexibility in most cases. This is explicit in the Roman Catholic insistence that contradictory propositions cannot be simultaneously accepted, and that revealed truth formulated as dogma is not flexible. Toleration of other groups and variations in non-essentials are not the same as flexibility of doctrine.

Another aspect of flexibility is the definiteness with which con-

166

victions are formulated. Narrow definition gives the individual a simple choice of belonging or not. Lack of definition can be charged with anxiety for the individual.

A few examples are given of different types of family organization that may affect mental health work. There is discussion of the Hindu joint family system with its wide range of recognized kinship and community of family property. The system protects but may also frustrate the young. The Confucian family organization is more rigid and social role is explicitly defined. In the Jewish family, the accent is on interpersonal love, which determines social role. Islamic families regard authority as derived from the human father's position next to God.

Important distinctions can be made between families with a parent-oriented or vertical authority structure, and those with a sibling-oriented or horizontal structure and which may tend to fragment into 'nuclear' units.

One finds a difference sometimes in the content of what people, from time to time, think constitutes right and wrong. The age at which the difference between right and wrong is demonstrated to children is an important conceptual factor. Other factors are, variously, the individual's own identifications (guilt) and the collective identification (shame). Sexuality appears in different ways among concepts of right and wrong. To the Chinese sexuality appears mainly as an integral part of the parental role. Christians have had much conflict of view and anxiety about sex, possibly due to the warm affective style of the monogamous Christian family which has tended to increase the emotional intensity of sexuality as compared with the style of life of a polygamous or an extended family form.

A new aspiration may make unhealthy what has previously been regarded by society as mentally healthy. A judgment on the mental health of people must take account of the existence of aspirations within the group.

Attitudes to error also vary. An interesting comparison can be made between the Soviet tendency to liquidate the deviant individual and the current Chinese communist attempt to redeem him. Mental health work sometimes encounters resistance if efforts to cure a psychiatrically sick individual are regarded as the redemption of someone who is deviating from socially acceptable behaviour.

The various religions have characteristic attitudes towards suffering and death. With Christianity, although different emphases occur, both positive acceptance of suffering in order to bring good out of evil, and recognition of the duty of Man to share in the suffering of humanity can be found. The Confucian attitude places no positive value on suffering.

Mental health work needs also to allow for the universal medical aspiration to prevent suffering. Many societies attempt to protect children against knowledge of pain and death. One Indian community, in contrast, believes that the major purpose of life is suffering, and Hindus, generally, regard death as deliverance from the suffering of this world. There is fairly widespread agreement that some element of pain or suffering is necessary for complete human maturity.

Attitudes towards mental illness throughout history have almost universally been dominated by notions of demoniacal possession, which are still extant over most of the world. There have been historical trends also to emphasize, in turn, metaphysical causes of mental disorder, the individual's own life experiences, social factors, and, in recent years, psychobiological factors.

Similarities between the great religions and ideologies are only outlined in the discussion. There are at least four common streams of agreement in connection with the pursuit of health: the value of intellectual study; the renunciation of the things of the flesh; devotion in order to understand the mysteries; and the pursuit of health through action. There might also be wide agreement on the proposition that harmony between cognitive and affective life that leads to integrated control by the former, will promote mental health.

CHAPTER 3

Some Practical Implications

OUR next task is to consider some practical implications of undertaking mental health work in different cultures. Up to the present stage of our discussion, the changes which we are advocating by implication are all in one direction, towards the position of the modern 'West'. Inasmuch as the concepts of mental health that are being discussed here have arisen in the West, and in various forms are in process of spreading into most parts of the world, it is not surprising that in the initial stages the tide of change should flow in one direction only. However, it has now become important to ask if changes are not desirable also in other directions.

It appears to us that a number of assumptions are constantly being made, both in the course of this discussion and, more generally, when mental health topics are being considered. In Chapters 1 and 2, many assumptions have been made both about the nature of mental health and about the character of the various religions and ideologies, respectively. Especially, we have assumed a measure of common agreement about these matters in drawing upon the basic information that we have used.

We have stated in the Introduction that it would be an impossibly Herculean task for us to attempt to make a systematic or exhaustive representation of the great religions and ideologies. Moreover, we have not been able to find a way of dealing even with our limited material, in a strictly comparable manner. Instead we have presented a number of selected illustrations for discussion. We are well aware that this is unsatisfactory; and it is probable that in the case of all the religions and ideologies to which reference is made, readers will wish to quarrel with or add to many of the illustrations that we have used. No statement will earn unanimous agreement.

It is part of our definition of a 'great' religion or ideology, as used in this context, that it can provide for a wide spectrum of human needs. It is unlikely that all aspects of a particular religious system will be equally acceptable to all members. We have therefore used as illustrations mainly matters that have seemed to us to be true, for the most part, of the religion concerned, and also to contribute something distinctive to the discussion. We have referred in the Introduction to an additional correction that needs making in the case of Christianity in that the majority of those who have contributed to our discussions have been familiar with Christian ways of thought and values to the degree that many aspects of the Christian position have tended to be taken for granted rather than stated expressly.

It is important to bear in mind that many of the assumptions made by mental health workers have not actually been established as facts; and this is especially true of many of the assumptions made about family life. For example, it is generally assumed in the West that the nuclear family system in which the family is reduced in size to its smallest viable biological unit is 'better' than the extended family system; that is, better suited to the type of change and development that characterises industrializing societies.

As a corollary to this, both in the 'West' and in the 'East' it is widely assumed that an existing joint family system will inevitably break up when exposed to the impact of industralization and 'development'. That this prospect is anticipated with intense anxiety was demonstrated during the discussions of the First Asian Seminar on Mental Health and Family Life (Tsung-yi Lin, 1958). At this seminar, attended by representatives from seventeen Asian countries, it appeared to be a common assumption that the interpersonal relationships within a nuclear family are of the same quality as those within an extended family; that there are no compensating values in the former that might do something to offset the numerical loss entailed by break-up.

Some Practical Implications

The view is widely held, and not only in respect of nuclear families, that the mother is unquestionably the best person to have charge of her own child; and this is used as an argument against the practice of young women leaving the home in order to work. It is possible that this feeling is linked with the equally widespread assumption that there is an antithesis between the machine and spiritual values, i.e. that industrialization is bound to weaken or destroy the value system of the community; which belief may well be linked with the fears entertained about the loss of the extended family.

Other assumptions are more general: for example, in the West, the majority value action more highly than contemplation; the usual belief being that the former is better adapted to the conditions of life in the West. The belief that an active sex life contributes positively to good health commands widespread support in many cultures. Further, it is widely held to be desirable that people should marry and have children. Celibacy in many cultures appears to be regarded as either a state of special privilege and responsibility or, in other circumstances, of incompleteness or, even, immaturity.

Many assumptions are made about the standard of living. Perhaps everywhere in the West and very widespread in the East, too, a rise in the standard of living is regarded as an essential part, if not the aim, of progress. A rising standard of living is by no means universally regarded as a 'good', however. In some cultures the attitude is tinged with the fear that in a time of general prosperity the older values will become superseded, and that the outcome will be one of moral deterioration. This fear may be connected with the anxieties felt over family changes to which reference has been made above. In countries with a high standard of living already, two antithetical assumptions will often be observed, almost side by side. On the one hand a rising standard of living in less-developed countries will often be regarded as an economic threat. On the other hand, it is often regarded as essential for economic health that all countries should share in the tide of prosperity.

The first practical implication of undertaking mental health work across cultural boundaries is to consider whether anybody knows enough to attempt anything of the kind. Important though it is for mental health experts to recognize and acknowledge all the gaps in their understanding, in fact, circumstances have forced our hand in this matter. In these days of easy communication, mental health practices – clinics, counselling, public education, etc. – are being copied from country to country without due thought about cultural applicability. A second comment is that when each culture is taken at its present level it seems probable that much can be done within existing systems and without the application of new knowledge to improve the lot of the handicapped, the diseased, and other unfortunate people.

The history of public health amply shows the unwisdom of embarking on curative or ameliorative work while neglecting the preventive aspects. In regard to the last-named, it will be generally agreed that far more objectively validated knowledge is needed before the intercultural promotion of mental health can be undertaken with confidence on a wide scale. One main objective of the current discussion is to consider certain areas in which this new knowledge may be looked for, so that mental health workers can extend their aspirations from the limited aim of improving the lot of the handicapped at a current level of technical competence towards wider advance.

Whatever the state of background knowledge, it will probably be agreed that the concepts of mental health that are to be promoted must be such that the majority of the people to whom they are presented will understand them. Here, a lesson can be learnt from religion. Whether the religion be deistic, animistic, demoniacal, or ethical, it will have little influence upon human hopes, doubts, and fears unless the ordinary person knows and understands what he believes. If objective ways can be worked out by which the ordinary man and woman in each culture concerned can come to understand what is meant by mental health, then a step forward will have been made. But in order that such understanding may be achieved it will be necessary, first, for the existing beliefs to be correctly identified.

The Introduction of Change during Mental Health Promotion

The principles underlying success in attempts to alter cultural conditions in the interests of mental health, and the hazards of such attempts, are very important considerations for practical mental health work. This will be true of therapeutic work with individuals no less than of prophylactic work in the community. In both of these aspects of mental health work change has to be envisaged, whether of the individual or of society, or, as is most likely, interdependently in both (see Soddy, 1950; Mead 1955).

Studies of children's development through successive changes have indicated a number of important principles of successful individual adaptation. To name a few of these: the opportunity for and impulse to change should come at an appropriate period in the life history of the individual, and the rate of change involved should not be greater than the individual's capacity to adapt; change if not arising spontaneously from within should be introduced by an agency that already has an established relationship with the child; and the process of change should bring with it inherent satisfactions as well as extrinsic rewards for accomplished change.

Difficulties which may arise from the introduction of change in the interest of mental health can be illustrated, for example, by the resistance which psychotherapists frequently encounter among their patients to forms of treatment which they recommend. This may be a result of an inadequacy of the relationship between the therapist and the patient; or alternatively, the language in which the suggestion is couched is so alien to the patient that there is insufficient mutual understanding for the change to be acceptable to the latter.

The induction of change in a community may be subject to conditions not unlike those which obtain in the case of the child: conditions of appropriateness of period, rate of change, relationships, and satisfactions. This possibility needs to be considered by Western-trained mental health workers who, when wishing to bring about change in a community in the interests of mental health, have a persistent tendency to interfere with child-rearing practices in that community. It is always instructive and sometimes salutary for mental health workers to investigate in detail the extent to which their formulations will actually be incorporated in the child-rearing practices of the mothers themselves. As one experienced British public health nurse expressed it: 'We tell the mothers that they must do this and that, but I think that in fact they do pretty much as they feel they want to, and perhaps it is better that they should!' Perhaps an important objective of this present study is to help mental health workers to develop techniques in their work that go beyond the offering of advice and the giving of instructions, into the promotion of understanding among the people with whom they are working.

Possible Disturbances arising from Change of Family Patterns

Much work has been done in the mental health field on child-rearing practices and interpersonal relations within the family. It may often happen that mental health workers will want to suggest various modifications in the interrelationships between parents and children, and husband and wife. Such desired changes may not be in accord with the existing family structure, which, in its turn, is interwoven with the religious system. The degree to which family and religious structure are interwoven, then, is a matter of great importance especially at times when family patterns are changing. For example, it would be difficult to introduce Western types of egalitarian attitudes to family relationships in an orthodox Islamic society.

The point can be illustrated, also, from the example of the many Muslims who come to the United States and lose connection with their religion, whether because they have no opportunity for religious observance, or because of a different structure of the family and a different attitude towards the father that is characteristic in the U.S.A. Whatever the religious and cultural background of the immigrant, if the original society had been one where there was great respect for the position of the parent, the U.S.A. would present to him a great social contrast; and in those cases in which the younger generation was educated and the older generation was uneducated, there would be conflict. Whether that conflict would strengthen the individual's religion or destroy it is an important question.

In advocating change in a culture other than his own, the mental health worker needs to ask himself questions of the order of: 'Are we introducing notions which come from the Western world, which influence the position of children, and which threaten to undermine the order of society and to produce conflict?'

Reference has been made above to the political stability resulting from the rigid Hindu caste system, and to the remarkable absence there in the past of organized political reaction from the underprivileged classes of the population.

We understand that during the last few years many changes have occurred in India, partly as a result of social changes during the Second World War, and it has been stated, though this is a matter of impression rather than exact ascertainment, that these have been accompanied by more ill-health and neurosis in families. But it would be misleading to say that the social changes have been responsible for the disorders. Rather, it may be that people are more and more coming to conceptualize the system as wrong, and to begin to move towards emancipation. Thus, matters that have hitherto been accepted as the natural order of events have increasingly come to be experienced by the people as frustration, with its concomitant stress effects.

There can be enormous differences in the way that these things will work out in practice; and movements towards change may encounter many obstacles in the great moral and religious principles of cultures. This can be illustrated in the question of salvation or enlightenment. According to Buddhist doctrine, enlightenment can be achieved by only the very few. In some religions salvation is not available for the ordinary person, though many religions will allow for a process of purification such as that in the Hindu doctrine of Karma. In some other religions the possibility of salvation may be restricted, for example, to men only, and the degree to which the possibility of salvation will apply to the lower sections of the population, socially and economically, will also vary very widely. For example, the Buddhist doctrine is generally not for women, though in other respects Buddhism provides outlets for normal human needs. Christianity teaches that since all men have been redeemed, salvation is for all, provided only that each takes the right means to achieve it.

In various sects and in some religions, rigid restrictions are put on the possibility of salvation, which may be only attainable through election by God, or alternatively by subscription to a narrow form of creed and practice, without which no salvation is possible.

One lesson to be learned from this by mental health workers is that in a religious atmosphere in which change for the better is a privilege severely restricted to a priestly caste or other limited social groups, a popular movement towards change can be stimulated only after preliminary steps have been taken to create among underprivileged people a climate favourable to change, which will include, among other things, a belief that change is not only desirable but possible.

'Vulnerability' to New Ideas

It will be an important part of the spread of mental health work to study in what ways established beliefs may be 'vulnerable' to new ideas. There have been in history many examples of behaviour and customs that enjoyed the sanction of religion, perhaps for centuries, and that have disappeared under the impact of certain new ideas to which they have become exposed, ideas that we might identify as being in line with mental health principles. Some of the best examples of this have been related to the principle of respect for human life. We would cite again the practice of cannibalism which has never withstood the exposure of the community concerned, to ideas of human worth; and this statement might be held to apply also to such practices as human sacrifice, slavery, the selling of female children, the exposure of girl babies, the killing of old people, and polygamy; though, in the case of some of the above, and especially the last-named, the inertia of social change has resulted in retention of the practice for as long as centuries after the tide of change has set in. It may be said, and notwithstanding any retrograde social innovations that may occur in a society in a time of crisis, that societies that have had any of the above-named social institutions in the past will not, without paying a severe price, go back to them after having been introduced to ways of life in which they are taboo.

A social scientist advanced the question as a speculative illustration whether, today, the entire Moslem world may not be 'vulnerable' to new ideas in relation to the improved status of women. There is a spreading desire among Moslem women to secure the status that is now general among Christian women. This, it may be felt, will give a good lead into mental health work among Moslem women, especially in relation to maternity and child welfare, where the women's role is dominant.

In one of our conferences the example was discussed of strict Buddhist life with its philosophy of non-attachment to which, it appears, even young mothers may subscribe; though the women are in general less identified with the philosophical system than are the men. The whole system may prove 'vulnerable' to notions of spontaneity in interpersonal relationships, such as are found among mental health values, today. It seems possible that a system of mental health that encouraged spontaneity in mother-child relationships might enjoy considerable advantages in such conditions.

The Mental Health Worker and Cultural Understanding

The argument that it is better for patient and therapist to have a common cultural background deserves further examination.

Let us take an example from a country from which professional people in many walks of life have been accustomed to going abroad for university and technical training. Nigeria and Thailand would be relevant examples, at different levels of industrialization. It will often happen that a psychiatrist who has gone abroad for training and who has returned home will engage in the treatment of a patient who has never left the country; or alternatively, a therapist who has been trained at home will treat a patient who has received his professional training abroad. In both instances there will probably be a wide, if superficial, cultural gap between patient and therapist and there will be some social and economic distance, also. On going back to cultural origins, however, it is possible to find fundamentals which will be common to both parties. The patient can still refer back to his historical background and find a common premise with the therapist.

Examples of a similar common premise can also be given from the Sudan, where, according to our information, it is considered very important in the culture that the primordial ideas that are characteristic of the indigenous system of medicine should be accepted by the doctor, even if trained in Western medicine, as well as by the patient. This importance has been brought home by a study of the various methods of interpretation of dreams that are employed. There is an ancient system of dream interpretation that is based on the Koran and which now has the official sanction of religion. For instance, the Koran frequently mentions women as gems, and a gem in a dream may come to mean a woman. There are also sayings of the Prophet which have a bearing on the interpretation of dreams. The fact that these primordial ideas and ancient traditions are part of the common background of both patient and doctor is important in making the most of psychological treatment. The doctor will interpret the dreams of the patient according to the Koran and the sayings of the Prophet rather than from the Freudian or other esoteric system of dream interpretation.

On the other hand, although mutual identification may give, among other things, a similarity of intuition, this may not be wholly advantageous to the course of treatment, because of the possibility of an important degree of emotional interference with the transference situation.

For example, an English child psychiatrist remarked that he had sometimes been conscious of getting on rather better with the treatment of some children from orthodox Jewish homes, than with some from ordinary English homes. It is possible that intuitive similarity may also bring with it certain emotional identifications and attitudes that impair understanding. In those cases where the cultural similarity is too great, the child might over-identify the doctor with its father or mother, or both. It would be very easy for the child to ascribe to the doctor attitudes which might belong properly to a dominant father, and so on; and although this might provide valuable material for interpretation, it would undoubtedly complicate the handling of the transference. In the case of some children from orthodox Jewish families, the transference situation might be more easily handled by a non-Jewish psychiatrist, who will not be so easily and so strongly identified by the child with a dominant father. Such identification may in some circumstances more than outweigh in disadvantages whatever is gained from cultural similarity.

In our experience, the above example has a much wider application than merely to relationships between Jews and Gentiles, and the whole question of cultural distance between patient and doctor deserves much more study than it has yet received. Although the sharing of a culture in common will, no doubt, be accepted as an important factor in communication between doctor and patient, and although our example of emotional interference from cultural similarity should not be allowed to obscure the importance of a common background, there may well be something of the order of an optimum degree of cultural difference between therapist and patient, about which it is important to know more.

One result of experience of the introduction of mental health work to places where it has not been seen previously is a clearer understanding that the mental health worker needs to know a very great deal about the conditions and circumstances of the society concerned. For example, it seems probable that the mental health worker needs to know very much more than is commonly known today about the values and the qualities of interpersonal relationships that exist in family structures belonging to cultures that differ from his own. It is partly a question of becoming able to bring into the mental health spectrum the highest values which religious and cultural ideologies have to offer. Without adequate knowledge, the danger facing mental health work will be of arriving at merely a kind of common denominator of values. Many people today, and probably in all religions and ideologies, suffer from a kind of value deprivation that prevents them from attaining the highest level of development and maturity to which their religion and ideology can bring them. It appears to us that a not dissimilar value deprivation can overtake mental health work that is not related to the high values of the culture in which it is being undertaken.

The Private Beliefs of Mental Health Workers

It is natural that mental health workers should have values of their own, both in regard to their profession and to their personal lives, that they regard as important and that they may be tempted to believe are universal. Care must be taken that such values are not developed into something which could assume its own kind of authority.

Granting that certain values are necessary to all individuals, and granting that many will need some way of putting themselves in touch with God, the point remains: Who should help the individual to do this? Should this be a function of the mental health worker; or should there be a division of labour, so that demands are not made on the mental health worker which he may not be able to satisfy? In many cases in present circumstances, no division of labour is possible because the personnel do not exist, and where such is the case an important further question may arise. What would be the effect if religious leaders of the community should wish to probe the value systems of people engaged in mental health work, in order to make sure that the latter were moving people in the direction acceptable to the religious leaders? What complications would such an attempt bring in its train?

What is the position of the individual mental health worker who, though not irreligious, yet subscribes to no religious system; and of the humanistic atheist? Need such mental health specialists be concerned with human values which verge upon the religious?

One view is that the problem can be solved if the mental health worker is a good man. If he is a good man he will devote himself to the cure of the mental illness and to giving the individual something to help to make his life more worth while. If a psychiatrist does not feel able to deal with the problem all the way, he can call on a more experienced and wise person within the field of the acknowledged values of the patient.

In cases in which the patient's religion is a clearly defined and important factor in the treatment situation, the point at which the therapist would call in the religious counsellor depends upon the experience of the therapist and upon his degree of personal identification with the patient's religion. In our view, the degree of responsibility that the therapist takes for the spiritual li.e of his patient is an integral part of the doctor-patient relationship.

In the converse cases in which the patient is agnostic, atheistic, or humanistic, the question of spiritual counselling may become very difficult indeed, but cannot be separated from the doctor-patient relationship any more than in the case of the religious patient.

Respect for Patients' Values

Let us consider the position of the doctor who does not share his patients' beliefs but, nevertheless, regards the beliefs of his patients as important to the latter.

In the course of discussion the question was raised of the position of a therapist who may be in general religious sympathy with one of his patients but not with another. The therapist, it is assumed, scrupulously respects his patients' beliefs, as a matter of principle, and regards them as of great importance to the patient. Would the difference between the two situations described make any difference in terms of therapy?

We have considered on pp. 177–80 some effects of cultural or ideological identification between therapist and patient. In a converse situation, one in which the two parties are opposed in a major degree to each other's beliefs, the empathy that is necessary for a successful therapeutic relationship might be, and probably would be, seriously impaired. If, for example, the therapist had a rooted conviction that there is nothing in the universe other than physical matter, and the patient an equally rooted conviction that matter is secondary in value to most other things, therapeutic empathy might well be stillborn, in which case a sterile treatment situation could result.

Some therapists consider that therapy can never be strictly non-directive, because it must always involve an empathic relationship with the patient. According to this view, in a successful treatment situation the therapist must inevitably affect his patient's scale of values and perhaps effect a change in his behaviour pattern. In these circumstances the effect of the therapist's lack of respect for the patient's values, when this is the case, is a matter of great moment.

It would be a natural consequence of these arguments that, for success, the therapist needs some degree of identification with the value system of the patient; and if carried to a logical conclusion it would follow that, for example, a Buddhist psychiatrist should treat only Buddhist patients.

On the other hand, and apart from the possible disadvantages of too great cultural similarity, it could be argued that this need not be so, because there is a common ground of human nature between, let us say, a Jewish doctor and a Gentile patient, which, apart from matters concerning religious denomination, is a positive link between them. Both may believe in the existence of God; and in the rightness of being good and the goodness of being right. Such common ground might be conducive to empathy.

Threat to Central Cultural Values

What happens in rapidly changing cultures when central values are threatened? One of the hazards of rapid change is the blurring of the focus of values that may occur; and it can be disturbing and disorienting for an individual to go from a society with a clear focus to one in which a focus is lacking.

> Our discussions also touched upon the question of rigidity and flexibility of identity. When identity is rigid it is hazardous to remove a centre of values, as has often been seen in the process of urbanization of Africans and others. Loss of the support of older identifications will often result in a very great increase in anxiety and insecurity. Thus the people will tend to lose the benevolent aspects of their old religions, without necessarily becoming positively identified with the benevolent aspects of the new order. Fear and guilt over the loss of old values will make them susceptible to the phylogenetically archaic elements of the new order, a tendency which is often increased by the accentuation of fear through the practice of malevolent religion and sorcery derived from the old religion. The dangers of loss of the focus of values have been realized, also, during the process of transformation of a peasant society into a proletariat.

The lesson is clear that in all change that is undertaken in the interests of mental health, the position of the integrated set of values of the society concerned must be protected.

Psychiatric Treatment and Ethics

Two aspects of the ethics of therapy can be discussed with profit here: first, how far it can be ethically justifiable to compel a non-volitional patient to have psychiatric treatment; and, secondly, how far it is possible to justify, on mental health grounds and in the interests of treatment, behaviour which is forbidden or disapproved of in the religion of the patient.

First, we discussed the question of coercion of the non-volitional patient, which will occur most commonly in connection with admission to a mental hospital. In Western society it has been usual to justify such coercion, roughly in this historical order, on one or more of three grounds: the protection of the community; the protection of the sick individual himself; and the securing of proper treatment for the individual (see also pp. 153–5).

Most Western societies are inclined to regard the mentally sick person has having been set outside the social group by the fact of his mental illness. It is unusual for normal people to continue to feel 'at one with' a psychotic member of the community. Most societies have some explicit way of segregating and depriving the psychotic individual of his civil rights and even of his liberty. At the same time, in many societies it is recognized that there are tendencies in the individual towards the regaining of health when it is lost, and which make morally imperative some attempt to reintegrate the sick individual with the group.

The explicit objectives of therapy in the case of mental illness will therefore include the arrest of the disorder, the reintegration of the patient's mental processes, and aid to the patient to gain insight and to regain membership of his social group. In Western societies such objectives are usually considered justification for the compulsory application of treatment, whatever the patient's resistance and to whatever degree it is recognized that compulsion may increase the trauma of the sick person's situation.

In a society in which a high value is set on the recovery and reintegration of the mentally sick individual, the use of force, deceit, or sharp practice within the law in order to secure the patient's admission to hospital with a minimum of disturbance will usually be accepted as the lesser of two evils. Society also will condone the patient's loss of liberty, even though individual liberty may be one of its highest values; and in many cases will show reluctance to restore civil rights even after the patient has regained insight.

In any measure to introduce to a society new forms of psychiatric treatment for non-volitional patients, great care needs to be exercised in order to establish hospital admission procedures that are ethically acceptable. Treatment proposals made with the best of intentions can be negatived by the arousal of public hostility.

The difficulty and delicacy of this situation are not always fully appreciated by those who are identified with the attempt to introduce a 'good thing' (i.e. therapy) to people whom they believe to be in need of help. This consideration is of such immense importance to the whole question of the treatment of the mentally ill that we shall take it up again in the light of the discussion of false analogies of the therapeutic process.

In the discussion on pp. 152–5 we have mentioned the question of so-called 'brain-washing' by Chinese communists and have noted that its objective appears to be reclamation of one who stands outside (communist) society, rather than liquidation. In the case of the Chinese communists it is clear that the captors and their society condone the use of force or deceit in order to get the prisoner into the concentration camp. While there, the prisoner will be subjected to such influence as his captors may think useful in order to get him to see the 'error of his ways'. When he has confessed his deviation, or – in the view of his captors – gained insight into his errors, and when they consider him fit, the prisoner will be released and, subject to close scrutiny, may be restored to a place in society.

We have concluded above (pp. 153–5) that in the case of religious conversion, one and the same process may appear to the protagonist as a matter for rejoicing, but to the antagonist as one for sorrow. In the case of political conversion that we have taken, 'brain-washing' appears to opponents as a wash-

ing away of a person's highest values, a corruption, but to
its proponents as a purification.

The term brain-washing has, we have noted, been applied
with unfortunate connotations to psychotherapeutic practice
by those who are hostile to it. We consider that the lesson
of this needs to be taken to heart by all who are responsibile
for securing psychiatric treatment for non-volitional patients.
The use of compulsion or deceit will almost certainly appear
to those who are unfriendly to or frightened of the aims of
psychotherapy, to be wicked. However well intentioned the
therapist, there are great dangers, in such potential attitudes,
to the success of any psychotherapeutic attempt.

Our illustration has been introduced as a strong warning
against the dangers of the unconscious introduction of the therapist's private ethical judgments into psychiatric practice. It is
extremely important to bear in mind the values of the people
most closely concerned, and to give full weight to the moral
relationship of ends and means in psychotherapy. Among the
matters that have to be given very earnest consideration are the
following: (*a*) the safeguarding of the ordinary human rights of
the individual during the period of mental illness; (*b*) the extent
of the responsibility for the mentally sick person to be assumed
by guardians and therapists; (*c*) the problem of the patient's
'presumed consent' to treatment – the validity of the assumption
that if he were not mentally ill he would wish, in the circumstances of illness, to be given treatment; (*d*) the problem of
professional confidence, and to what extent information gained
confidentially can be used in the supposed interests, but not with
the consent, of the non-volitional patient; (*e*) the length to which
the therapist can go in order to attain an end to which he but
not his patient can subscribe.

Psychosurgical operations will be of particular concern in this
last connection, e.g. the operation of prefrontal leucotomy (lo-
botomy) which is sometimes prescribed for the relief of certain
conditions of severe intractable anxiety, depressive states, etc.
It appears to have been established that the operation may in

some cases impair the patient's capacity to make judgments. This raises the extremely important question of what are the criteria that the psychiatrist will need to observe in advocating treatment that has a known risk of disturbing the patient's moral relationships?

Responsibility and Anxiety

Another aspect of the ethics of therapy is the anxiety that the individual may experience if he should have to choose between taking or not taking a course of behaviour that is forbidden by his own religious group but which, he understands, will relieve him of anxiety.

It has been represented to us that during the course of psychotherapy it may happen that a patient will adopt a course of action that is in conflict with values that have been important to him; and that such action may be recommended by the therapist. We have many reservations about the justification of making such recommendations in the name of therapy, but we have to admit that the situation does arise in practice, and that the patient's subsequent behaviour may have originated in the therapeutic situation.

It may possibly happen that a patient will be faced with a decision whether or not to take a course of action that is in conflict with his convictions but which he sincerely believes may lead him towards mental health. The patient will not adopt the course of action if his convictions represent for him a higher value than mental health.

This situation which, we believe, arises less commonly than is often supposed, deserves brief discussion. From the Roman Catholic point of view, for example, and no doubt from that of other Christian denominations also, we understand that such an issue would probably be determined on the principle: 'For what shall it profit a man, if he shall gain the whole world, and lose his own soul?'

There is a variety of situations that might be associated with this kind of problem; e.g. questions of contraception, marital separation, divorce, and remarriage; or masturbation; or attempted suicide; or some questions of obedience to authority.

From a Roman Catholic viewpoint, we are informed, conflict might arise between moral principle and a course of action which the patient has come to believe is in the interest of his mental health. He might be faced with the choice of what he regards as a lesser good, mental health, at the expense of his moral well-being. He may not choose an immoral means in order to achieve mental health. Apparent conflicts of this kind are complicated in practice and tempered by other considerations. Thus the very state of mental health of the patient, and his level of maturity or immaturity, are relevant in assessing his responsibility.

In the Roman Catholic view it has always been acknowledged that a human act is influenced by and can be removed from rational control by the operation of the passions. In addition, it appears that among the more rigid systems of religious morality, definitions of moral responsibility tend to be changed under the impact of notions derived from psychiatry. For example, the idea of compulsive behaviour now widely acceptable in the West, would not have been understood in the same psychological terms three hundred years ago.

In cases of conflict between religious morality and psychotherapeutic desiderata, the resolution of the conflict lies in a proper understanding by both sides of the viewpoint of the other. Under these conditions it seems likely that areas of serious misunderstanding may be narrowed.

The Mental Health Worker and the Minister of Religion

It will be advantageous to consider more particularly what division of function might be made between the mental health worker and the minister of religion. A division of labour is both sensible and practical; it is impracticable to think of the expansion of the mental health movement without specialization of such functions.

Moreover, as we have seen above, the possibility of incompatibility between courses of action advocated by a mental health worker and a minister of religion, respectively, is sufficiently great to warrant consideration of the best ways in which harmful clashes can be avoided.

This problem can arise no less during counselling than during therapy. An illustration can be taken from the field of marriage problems, from a case in which both parties have come to the conclusion that their marriage relationship is insupportable. A Roman Catholic marriage counsellor, we are told, might in such a case conclude that the marriage situation, as presented, is incompatible with the full mental health of both parties. His attitude might be expressed as follows: 'You may not divorce, in the sense of breaking the marriage bond, and having the right to marry again. You might consider separation. If you separate, you may be happier, and indeed, mentally healthier. But you should consider also your spiritual welfare and that of your children. You must make the choice. Which is more important in your eyes – your own mental health or the spiritual welfare and mental health of your children?'

The dilemma facing the non-Catholic mental health worker is no less subtle. He may come to the conclusion that, in the case cited, divorce was a necessary solution to an intolerable situation; but he would also say that divorce could not be regarded as other than a failure in human relationships. In other words, divorce would leave the essential mental health problems of the couple unsolved. This dilemma can be solved only in relation to the hierarchy of values of the persons concerned.

While conceding the need for some separation of the functions of mental health worker and of minister of religion, we would stress that the mental health worker, so far as is possible, should be familiar with the culture and religions of the people among whom he works. It would help if, with their psychiatric training, mental health workers were given training concerned with the wide spectrum of values that exist in their community.

It is unreasonable in this context to demand that only one party to this proposed collaboration should undertake a certain amount of personal preparation in the field of competence of the other party. If a division of labour is to have any validity, it is equally important for the minister of religion to have a comparable familiarity with principles of mental health.

There is, in our opinion, a third party whom it is important to include in this proposed collaboration, that is those people in society who are attempting to do something of the work of ministers of religion and mental health workers without the orientation of either of the professional trainings. We refer to the thousands who are working in youth movements and similar aspects of social service. Many such movements are already under religious auspices. We would advocate the attachment also of mental health workers familiar with the religious concepts, values, and beliefs of the people concerned, so that mental health principles may, in time, permeate their activities.

It was stated in one of our background papers that, 'Mental health is one of the most important conditions which make possible the realization of idealistic aspirations, but is not an aspiration itself. Moreover, the mental health worker, at least in principle, never propagates ideals as such, or systems, or solutions of human problems.' However, during the course of our discussions we have taken the view that mental health can be an aspiration itself and, further, it could be suggested that the mental health worker's function is to propagate the solution of human problems by scientific techniques, at a natural level. It is not the formal function of religion to produce mental health. Similarly, it is not the normal function of a mental health worker to produce the perfect human being. As we have discussed above, there can be situations in which the mental health worker's techniques will promote mental health in an individual whom the religious teacher can lead on to his concept of salvation. In the case of the individual who has a scrupulous state of mind about moral issues it is difficult to decide in practice how far his problem may be a religious one. The psychiatric worker is equipped to deal with one sector of experience of the human being; but it is rare for a problem to be solely that of mental illness. If a dual role could be combined of understanding of the person's mental health and of his religious problems, difficulties would be fewer, but there still may be transference complications when one individual has to play a dual role. Even if he happens to be doubly trained, the therapist who has patients from many denominations or different religions may find that it is not helpful to undertake both roles. When the therapist encounters a religious problem during the course of treatment it may often be better to discuss with the patient the advisability of calling in the aid of the appropriate minister, priest, pastor, rabbi, guru, imam, or counsellor. This might apply both during the course of treatment and at the termination, when the therapist might feel that he had gone about as far as was possible and that the remainder of the problem lay in the field of religion.

We would make a strong plea for more institutionalized and more formal co-operation between mental health workers and ministers of religion; for closer working together and more overlap of understanding on both sides. As we have already remarked, it would be a good thing to have more ministers of religion with greater knowledge of mental health, and more mental health workers with a better understanding of religious issues.

The difficulty of making a demarcation between a mental health and a religious function may be very great indeed, when that stage in the transference situation is reached where the therapist's own convictions become a matter of moment in the treatment.

We have referred above (pp. 183–7) to the ethical considerations involved in securing treatment for the non-volitional patient, i.e. when the therapist considers that the patient needs treatment. The problem of the therapist's own convictions, when it arises during treatment, is more subtle and in many ways may be even more difficult. It may be possible to generalize that it is rarely helpful to the patient for the therapist to conceal the existence of his own convictions. Although the prevailing mood of the therapist will probably be one of scrupulous respect for the current convictions of the patient, there may be occasions when the therapist will conclude that the patient's conviction is symptomatic of his difficulty and it may be the therapist's duty not to stand strictly one one side. Moreover, it may equally be the duty of the therapist to take great care not to substitute his own value system for that of his patient, under the guise of treatment.

Specialization of Mental Health Workers' Functions

Specialization of functions has been discussed as arising out of the bigger issue of whether mental health is to be regarded as an ultimate value or an instrumental value. We need now to go on to discuss who shall do what. Even if it is recognized that the mental health worker has a specialized role, it is important not to prevent the worker who is capable of taking more than one role from doing so. But, on the other hand, it is no less important, in this field, to ensure that science does not become a value that is exclusive to the mental health worker. There is a possibility, if science only is emphasized, for workers to become over-professionalized and cut off from other human values.

Mental health workers who have come from a less sophisticated society, who obtain training of the industrialized Western type and then practice in more traditional culture conditions, will have some problems of personal attitude to solve. They 'will probably have an urge to change matters; but they may gradually feel that in order to develop psychiatry it is necessary to build on a foundation of harmony with and understanding of the community. It may be felt that in a community which has deep roots in religious healing, it is important not to act in a competitive way, but rather in a supplementary manner. The role of the psychiatrist will be different in various countries.

In the Sudan, for example, we understand that the psychiatrist tends to be regarded as a medicine man, or as a sort of religious healer, and it is possible there to interpret to the patient his own symptoms in accordance with his own traditional though processes (p. 178). Similarly the treatment can be guided along the traditional system of thought. Psychiatrists would have found it far more difficult to start their work in the Sudan had they not felt the need to work through the religious teaching.

Utilization of Available Skills

The urgency of bringing help to people who are suffering will transcend the niceties of professional qualification. In no country are there sufficient numbers of trained workers available, and in many countries there are practically none. There are, however, many other possible resources, such as those to be found in religious circles; but in seeking for support for therapeutic endeavour it should be borne in mind, once again, that religion is not to be regarded primarily as instrumental to mental health, nor therapy primarily as an instrument of religious purposes.

In one of our background working papers it was stated, 'He [the mental health worker] tries to give help and assistance, based on science, with scientific knowledge of man and his drives.' In principle this is true, but it is not possible for all mental health workers to be trained in scientific method and concepts, and the best use must be made of available skills in people. Conversely, the investment of different roles in the mental health worker will vary a great deal from culture to culture. Scientific training does not necessarily mean that the worker is capable. Psychotherapy is not an entity in itself, but a systematic differentiation of knowledge of something which starts as a direct human contact. It also has an intimate and organic relationship to conditions in the social order.

The aims and objectives of people in the social work field are bound to vary in relation to the explicit mental health objectives: for example, maternity and child welfare workers cannot escape a mental health role. It might be said that the preliminary qualifications of the mental health worker are that he has some conceptualization of mental health as an aspiration and some perception of a way to achieve it. The question of scientific training is of another order.

SOME SPECIFIC CONDITIONS AFFECTING MENTAL HEALTH WORK

During the course of our discussions we have encountered a number of illuminating examples of specific conditions that may be encountered during the course of mental health work which it may be helpful to describe.

Brahmin Rigidity

A discussion took place of the case of a young Brahmin who, as commonly happens, returns to his father's house in a disturbed state after an absence, during the course of which he has done many things forbidden to a strict Brahmin (pp. 141–3). According to our Western-trained Brahmin psychiatrist informant, he will not be accepted by his (orthodox) family. His father would regard him as delinquent, although a psychiatrist might regard his disturbed state as neurotic. Many Hindus of the Indian regiments who had served abroad during World War I were made out-caste in this way on their return to India, and caste women refused to marry them because they had gone overseas, eaten foreign meat, and drunk water 'polluted' by the touch of Christians. It appears that after World War II, although far more Brahmins had gone overseas on war service than during World War I, a similar situation did not arise to anything like the same extent as previously, and this may be regarded as evidence of a wide movement of change.

A Religious Vow mistaken for Psychosis

A striking incident was reported involving a Moslem woman student at a Western university, who decided to fast for three days before attempting some extremely difficult scientific work. She asked a friend, who was a Hindu, to see that she

194

was not disturbed while fasting. During that time she would not eat, drink, move, or talk. At 2 a.m. on the first night an American in the same group became alarmed because of the student's refusal to speak, eat, or drink, and a psychiatrist was called in. The friend who had undertaken to see that the student was not disturbed had obviously become frightened, and because it was erroneously believed that she, too, was a Moslem, the psychiatrist concluded that the cause of the behaviour was not religious, but rather a mental disturbance. Schizophrenia was suspected. To add to the circumstances prejudicing consideration of the case, the Hindu friend had been a psychiatric nurse, so that she looked at her from a psychiatric, not a religious point of view. So it happened that the girl was sedated and sent to the disturbed ward of a mental hospital.

While in the disturbed ward, in the presence of several doctors, the student later said, 'Do you remember the way a host treats a guest and the way in which the host and guest relate only to each other? When one is fasting one is related only to God and not to other people.' In fact, the student went through several years of most difficult work and at the end of it wrote an excellent book. This was a case of consistent misinterpretation, in which the first image distorted subsequent interpretations.

Sudden Emergence from Protection

Possible traumatic effects of exposure to abrupt change are illustrated by the case of a certain Indian girl who was studying medicine in Europe. When she started taking lectures on psychiatry during the fourth year, she developed various minor hysterical symptoms, and suddenly went into a severe anxiety state. Her contention was that her anxieties were due to the fact that she had been in purdah (the traditional protected life of women in orthodox Indian Moslem society) until she was seventeen and had come straight from it to an open society. Twelve months later it was clear that her anxiety was due not so much to this sudden release from

purdah as to an inability to relate to anyone among her
fellow students. There were other Indians in the group who
had adjusted adequately to Western life, whereas she had
not. Although in all outward respects she was a Westernized
Indian, the cause of her inability to relate to others lay much
deeper in her personality than her sudden coming out of
purdah.

However, it is true that coming out of purdah at the end
of adolescence can be a traumatic experience. Had the girl
come out of purdah in India before going abroad her anxiety
might not have been as intense. Our attention has been
drawn to cases of Indian men students in London complain-
ing of delusions and of hearing voices. They were not used
to English conditions of life and to living in lodgings. Some
of them, although they could speak English, could not understand what English people were saying. They were in a state
of severe depression, had frightening dreams and would
awake in the middle of the night and disturb other people in
the lodging-house. Previously they had lived very sheltered
lives under the care of their parents, and then suddenly had
to face an entirely different set of circumstances.

We are informed that one curious effect can be seen
among some members of the new generation of Islamic young
women when they no longer wear the veil. It appears that
the face is still a focus of great sensitivity. Young women in
the universities tend to be bashful and shy, because, apparently, the face is a vulnerable part of the body to them. It
will be interesting to see whether the next generation will get
over this.

In 1951–1954 a study was made of Nigerian students from
different social strata, in England. Colleagues from Africa
and England examined the cases of those who had broken
down psychologically and succeeded in fitting them into a
homogenous pattern of psychology. Subsequently, however,
after two years spent in tracing the families of these people
at home, it was found that over 90 per cent had histories of
earlier mental breakdown.

Nigeria – Dual Loyalties

An interesting problem of attitudes can be seen among members of strong sub-cultural societies in Nigeria, where some of the Christians take part regularly in ancestor-worship rituals. If they did not attend the rituals they might suffer from anxiety through fear that one of their children might die or something else might happen to them.

In the view of a Nigerian psychiatrist it would be justified to encourage such a man to go back to his people and carry out the rite, and his anxiety might be relieved in this way. Alternatively, a Western rational point of view could be advanced that the threat was producing guilt feelings in the man and that his anxiety was groundless. With sufficient time, the anxiety might be relieved in that way, also. The question arises which, to a psychiatrist and a scientist, would be the better role?

There appears to be no simple answer to this question. A psychiatrist whose desire is to preserve his country's institutions alongside the Western ways of life might well express his hope to the man concerned that the Church would not excommunicate or judge him adversely if he were to return to his own people and take part in the rituals. The psychiatrist might hold that this was not a case of a Christian giving his allegiance to other gods, but rather the preservation of something that was precious to the culture. A Western-trained Nigerian psychiatrist in fact expressed his belief that there is no tendency on the part of the churches and other Westernized institutions to discourage or stigmatize those who go back to their villages for rituals. We are also informed that this is expressly forbidden by some Christian missions. To some people, therefore, such reassurance will not be enough and it might be necessary to help them to overcome the need to go back.

From the side of the indigenous institutions there is tremendous encouragement for people to go back. Theirs is an ambitropic religion, people being able to take part in Christian religious activities and also the activities of the indigenous institutions. Western religious ideas are accepted by most people in a Western social contact. The mental health problems in relation to religion are wrapped up with the indigenous institutions. There is no fixed point in behaviour where the Nigerian society regards the individual as being no longer responsible but mentally ill; but according to our informant the point at which a man would be regarded as mentally ill is not very different from that in any other culture.

Values set on Boys and Girls

One of the conditions that a mental health worker must take into account is that not the same value may be set by the community upon girls as upon boys. For example, in India, the very big discrepancy between the number of adult males and females cannot be explained in terms of sex ratios at birth. The inferences from the statistics are that special care is given to the boy in the family and that the female children are not cared for with the same degree of solicitude. This differentiation might be unconscious, or it might be that medical care is sought more for the boy than for the girl. In India the situation is dramatically and tragically serious because many more girls die than boys.

A Hindu Brahmin psychiatrist has remarked that the equal treatment of children regardless of sex is laid down in the Hindu scriptures, but that there have been many changes during the last few centuries. Female children became neglected and were regarded as less important during the prolonged disturbed period of the Mogul invasions. The Hindu attitude when the fighting man went to battle was that they did not want to leave their women behind to be violated by the invaders or carried away as slaves. The custom grew up that the women had to kill themselves when they heard that their husbands had been killed. This led to the situation in which Hindu women considered widowhood as the worst form of suffering, and resulted in the practice of suttee or the ceremonial self-immolation of the widow on her dead husband's pyre.

To this view we would add the comment that for Hindu women to feel that the greatest evil is widowhood suggests that some more fundamental factor is operating than an historical fear of slavery. This indication of inferiority feeling in the case of women may relate also to the differential in the care that appears to be taken of boys as compared with girls.

Children's Experience of Death of Others

On page 160 we have discussed some attitudes to suffering, death, and the 'tragedy of life' that can be found among various peoples. These attitudes vary very widely but there is one particular attitude widely prevalent in the West about which a comment might be made from a psychiatric point of view.

We understand that in the United States it is quite usual in some circles for the children to be totally protected from any personal experience of the phenomenon of death. Very often the first intimate experience of the death of another person is the death of a parent, when they themselves are perhaps forty-five or fifty years of age. People in the United States are beginning to question whether shutting off children from death is not bad for their mental health, for they fail to participate in an experience which, nevertheless, they know exists. There are complaints at university level that it is difficult to teach classical literature to students who have not had any experience of the death of other human beings known to them. It is inconceivable that individuals will not have to face the fact of death at some point in their lives.

It may be that there are mental health principles about the way in which children should be introduced to the fact that living things, including human beings, die.

Mental Health and Value Systems

Intensity of Relationship

It is the usual experience that mental health work will involve the introduction of changes to the community as a whole, in the form of new services, new laws, and so on; and to individuals and families in various more intimate ways. The question of attitude to change is, therefore, important, because the mental health worker may best hope to succeed through the creation of a climate of opinion that is favourable to the kinds of change that are involved. To do this successfully will involve understanding of the styles of interpersonal relationships that characterize the various family forms in a community. It is legitimate to inquire into the possibility that a connection exists between attitudes to change in a community and the changes that individuals have experienced and undergone in the course of childhood development.

Among the many well-known forms of family organization that exist in different cultures and social variations within cultures, there are differences in the number of adults that come into contact with the young child and in the degree of intimacy that obtains in such contacts. An example can be given, on the one hand, of a family made up of the smallest biological unit of mother, father, and baby, on their own; and, on the other, of a family in which an extended range of adults is in daily relationship with the young child. Varations of this order, and intermediate forms, are found in human family life, and where a degree of cultural homogeneity exists there may be a significant prevailing style of interpersonal relationship in family life in the community.

A Western-trained child psychiatrist has suggested that where only one or two people have been involved in the care of a small child the intensity of the quality of the interpersonal relationships developed in that family may be greater than where a larger number of people have had to do with the child: and that this difference may be significant to the type of relationships that the child will build up (see also p. 130). If there is a significant degree of homogeneity of style among the families in a community, this suggested variation in quality of intensity of interpersonal relationships will be important to consider.

This suggestion should not be taken as implying that in a nuclear family all relationships are formed at a stronger intensity and in an extended family at a weaker intensity; but rather that, within these two types of family system the stage is set, as it were, for relationship formation at a higher and at a lower pitch of intensity, respectively, unless specific local conditions alter the circumstances.

To continue, it has been argued that in a nuclear family, in which the mother, father, and child form a closely knit unit, the adoption of change by a tiny baby depends upon the skill of the parental handling. For example, the mother helps the child to transfer the satisfaction that it has gained from sucking at the breast, to new attainments, of which the actual process of feeding itself is one example. The baby's attainment of new skills is a powerful source of mutual pleasure between mother and child and enhances their mutual relationship. This experience may create what might be termed a climate of acceptance of change, in that the introduction of change to the child in a warm affective setting may lead the child to have a positively accepting attitude, to be pleasurably stimulated by and to enjoy the satisfactions to be gained out of changing.

Subsequently, as the child becomes identified with its parents and with what it can appreciate of the parental value system, it develops beyond the state in which it gains satisfaction in doing new things for the sake of its mother, into a state of 'built-in' satisfaction in doing new things for the sake of the new things. Such a child has enhanced the positive attitude to change that it gained during infancy and finds satisfaction in the specific items of change. This satisfaction is a source of strength that may be characteristic of the intense form of interpersonal relationships that, as has been argued on theoretical grounds, may be fostered in the nuclear family.

On the other hand, in an extended family in which a young child may have half a dozen adults and many older children in its immediate circle, it is possible that interpersonal relationships are less intense than those which characterize a baby in the sole care of its mother. Change may be introduced to this child by any or all of the people around; and there is less likelihood that the baby's acceptance of change will enhance its relationship with any one key adult.

For the nuclear-family child in the care of a single adult, it is likely that the intimate details of the mother's behaviour to the child will become affectively toned for the baby. If six different adults are handling the baby in an extended family, the minutiae of its experiences will tend to lack specific character for the baby. Hence the affective response of the baby tends to be to a kind of 'highest common factor' of motherly care. In the earliest months the difference will not be great but it will increase as behaviour develops farther away from its early instinctual forms.

Thus it may be that in the extended family the 'highest common factor' of maternal behaviour assumes something of the importance in interpersonal relationships that the more specific intimate relationships will have in the nuclear family. In other words, the form of the family relationships may be more influential than their specific content.

This argument has been advanced in full recognition that the above generalization can apply only to the situation that tends to prevail in extended and nuclear families, respectively, and that what will actually happen in each family will depend on the reality situation there. However, if the generalization be accepted for purposes of discussion, it might be legitimate to infer that in the extended family there may be a 'built-in' tendency towards the maintenance of the form and structure of family organization and the continuation of its habitual modes of behaviour. In other words, the child growing up in a typical extended-family type of emotional relationships will gain satisfaction from maintenance of family patterns; whereas the child growing up in typical nuclear-family relationships will tend to find satisfaction in the actual process of changing and, particularly, in the evolution of interpersonal relationships.

The above theoretical speculation has a bearing on the mental health worker whose task it is to introduce change to a community or to individuals in the interests of mental health. If it be true that in a society structured around the nuclear family there is a tendency for people to find satisfaction in change itself and especially in change of style of interpersonal relationships, then a mental health worker would be best advised to seek to introduce change individualistically. On the other hand, in a society with an extended-family structure, it would be more promising to institutionalize the changes desired so that they became identified with traditional patterns of family relationship.

Another related aspect of the introduction of change in the interests of mental health has been touched on above (p. 173) in discussing differing patterns in family life. Where society is parent-oriented, the most fruitful approach might be linked with authority. Where society is sibling-oriented, the most effective approach would be dependent upon the effectiveness of the social institutions devised to control sibling rivalry and to deal with deposed figures of authority. In the case of the sibling-oriented society an authoritarian approach would be inappropriate and, when tensions related to authority figures remain unresolved, might be quite inimical to success.

In this field there is a need for more systematic study in order that appropriate approaches may be worked out for different types of society.

Forced Acceptance of New Values

It is important for the success of mental health work to consider the psychological trauma that might result from attempts to force people to accept new values. We have discussed immediately above some of the factors that affect the acceptance of change by society (see also p. 173). To recapitulate briefly some of these: change is most easily accepted by a community when the motive to change arises from within the community, and when the rate of change is not greater than the capacity of the society to respond to change. When a society is exposed to change through contact with other societies, it is sometimes acceptable, so that the society concerned becomes identified with the change. On the other hand, when change is forced upon a community against its will, it is probable that the change will become identified in the minds of the people with its alien origin. The natural result of this will be to invoke reactions that are appropriate to the alien source of change rather than to the change itself.

More than this, change imposed involuntarily from without will invoke defensive reactions typical of the social organization. Thus it might be argued from theoretical premises that in a society in which a 'nuclear' family type of intimate interpersonal relationships prevails, change coming from without might be more readily accepted if the affective relationship with the alien origin is positive; but if negative, rapid change might occur in a contrary direction. Where an 'extended' family type of inter-personal relationships prevails, change coming from without is more likely to be met outright with rejection and an increase in social rigidity.

It is important not to confuse rigidity and inflexibility with cultural strength; or flexibility and labile change, even in a contrary direction, with cultural weakness. If very strong changing influences are met by social rigidity, the ultimate result may be cultural breakdown. On the other hand, mobility in a contrary direction may have dangerous results, too.

The chief lesson of these theoretical considerations for mental health workers is that when change is forced upon a society from alien origins by the compulsion of circumstances, which is a common feature of the modern world, there are here some theoretical guides which may be of value in promoting mental health in the community in times of change. Again, there is a great need for more exact knowledge in this field.

Intuition

The Concise Oxford Dictionary defines intuition as 'immediate apprehension by the mind, without reasoning; immediate apprehension by sense; immediate insight'. Most observers of human behaviour regard intuition as very important for interpersonal human relationships, but also as being very variable between individuals as to quality and the amount to which it affects behaviour and communication.

It is possible to trace the development of intuition in the small child out of his exploratory experiences during the toddler period, but comparatively little is yet known about the process.

A British child psychiatrist made a speculation about the emergence of intuition in the child. He remarked that in the English cultural pattern, among others, it is usual for a child to learn certain important processes of interpersonal communication with its mother, e.g. of mood and attitude, at about the same time as it is beginning to gain understanding about movement in its immediate surroundings. Such understanding will rapidly become relegated to unconsciousness and will be transmuted into function automatically. The child will arrive at the state in which it can move around without giving conscious thought to the arrangement of the furniture or the stairs, for example, and will adapt automatically and with little conscious consideration to small changes in the material environment, alterations in daily routine (if this is flexible), and to minor changes in the mother's mood.

Such automatic appreciation of the situation and ready adaptation will depend upon a complicated system of communication which is built up in the child; a system that will include feedback between child and environment, and will also extend to the field of social relationships. Even at this early stage it bears a resemblance to that refined complex of qualities which we recognize as intuition.

The point can be illustrated further by taking the case of the child who has become oriented in the material environment, but who lacks social or interpersonal relationships; in whom social responsiveness has not become fully part of the automatic response system. This condition may be met clinically in various forms of what has been termed 'autism'. The autistic toddler child will remain preoccupied, even obsessed, with uncompleted exploration of the material world, which it never comes to understand fully, so that the link between the material world and human relationships is not forged. The child remains imperceptive in social contacts, and it is a matter of clinical experience that a seriously affected child will discover how to manage social relationships, if ever, only at a later age, through cognitive development.

It is evident that much of social conduct depends upon the intuition of the people concerned, and that therefore this should be regarded as an important area for further study.

Objectivity – Sympathy

It appears to us that sympathy between human beings may be a universal phenomenon, and in any interpersonal relationship a minimum of sympathy must exist before empathy can be established. Many people will make an antithesis between sympathy and objectivity of attitude, and may regard objectivity as a lack of sympathy. We do not accept this view. Sympathy may interfere with strict objectivity, but it is likely that objectivity without sympathy may not be truly objective because it may lead to distortions in the estimation of emotional values.

The discussion on this topic has included consideration of some aspects of empathy and intuition and their relationship to the sharing of a common culture which can make it easier for a therapist to communicate with a patient with whom he shares a culture (p. 177). This is the basis upon which, for example, a Roman Catholic patient and a Jewish doctor are able to communicate. Such a shared culture is not a matter of particular belief. When both parties belong to an overall culture, they can understand enough to communicate with each other; but if one comes from Europe and the other from Nigeria, for example, then communication will be more difficult. Communication will be more difficult still in the case of areas that are entirely different, such as New Guinea and many other parts of the world.

It may be that when all the cultures are considered together there might well be found a common element that could be called 'other-worldly', which would enable a therapist and a patient of markedly different culture to communicate with each other. On the other hand, in those not uncommon cases in which a therapist takes for granted a definition of the universe in completely material terms, he will flout important aspects of a relationship of a member of a group where the material world is defined quite differently.

It sometimes happens that when the doctor is being 'objective' the patient may be inclined to regard him as not sympathetic. If in being 'objective' the doctor is doing violence both to his feelings and to his intuitive methods of communication developed during the course of life's experience, the doctor's so-called objectivity can cause a lack of rapport with the patient and interrupt the communication between doctor and patient.

On the other hand, intuitive similarity is not wholly advantageous, since it may give rise to emotional interference with important factors in the therapeutic situation. An example of this was given on page 179, in the case of a Gentile psychiatrist and a Jewish child. If there is a wider degree of cultural variation involved, such unhelpful identifications are less likely to occur.

Rapport and Intuition

All therapeutic relationships are dependent in some degree on the establishment of rapport between patient and therapist. Rapport is a two-way relationship in which both sympathy and empathy can be prominent. The extent to which possession of the quality of intuition by the therapist is a necessary ingredient of the establishment of rapport is one of the great unresolved problems in the field of therapy.

Distinctions have been drawn between intellect and intuition since ancient times. The matter was discussed quite explicitly by the great eleventh-century Islamic physician, Avicenna, who said that intuition is superior to intellect; that in moments of intuition one can grasp reality in a single pulse. He maintained that there is a *rapport* between Nature and the mind, which is used in the patient-doctor relationship, and that the physician must have a sense of intuition to choose, pursue, and accomplish treatment.

We are looking for approaches which will have meaning to people coming from many different points of view and with different backgrounds. Knowledge that is totally dependent on intuition cannot be communicated from one person to another and cannot be checked by a second person, that is, unless routes of communication can be established.

Although intuition functions best between people who have some similarity of background, it is important to recognize that the art of attending to non-verbal cues, even in someone of a very different culture, can be learned. Our increasing knowledge of the importance of various types of body movement in interpersonal communication, and the extent to which such forms of communication are culturally stylized, suggests that they can be systematized and taught, as language can be taught. This is an important field of further exploration.

SUMMARY

A number of unproven assumptions concerning individual and family life are commonly made in mental health work; e.g. that the style of family life in which the worker was himself brought up is 'the best'; that the mother is always the best person to have charge of her own child; that there is an antithesis between machine and spiritual values. Assumptions of various kinds are also made about the active, in comparison with the contemplative, life; about sex and the desirability to procreate children; about the necessity to raise the standard of living, and so on.

Mental health changes need to be based upon principles known in the community, avoiding sudden change of family pattern, such as the abrupt introduction of an egalitarian attitude into a society with a parent-oriented family structure. Much can be learnt from the study of how the children of the community are exposed to change. In some societies, change itself is a privilege restricted to limited social groups, and in others, such as an orthodox Hindu society, little or no change is possible. The success of mental health promotion depends partly upon the creation of a climate favourable to change and a belief that change is desirable and possible.

Established beliefs and customs in society may be 'vulnerable' to new ideas, under certain conditions. Many practices (e.g. human sacrifice, slavery, and to some extent polygamy) do not survive in a society that is exposed to the different values of other societies. The improved status of women in many parts of the world appears to make a good opportunity for mental health work in countries where women still occupy an inferior status.

The mental health worker needs to have cultural understanding, but not necessarily cultural identification. As in the case of therapist and patients, so in that of the mental health worker, there may be an optimum degree of cultural distance, which may be no more than a class difference. At all events the mental health worker must know and respect the high values of the people with whom he works.

A division of responsibility between therapist and spiritual counsellor is advocated. Responsibility for the spiritual life of his patient is an important question in the doctor-patient relationship. The development of empathy depends to some extent on the therapist respecting the beliefs of his patients. With such respect, empathy can extend across wide religious differences, because of the common ground of human nature. Threat to the central values of an individual or community may increase anxiety and insecurity to a harmful degree.

Mental Health and Value Systems

It is important to guard against the unconscious introduction of the therapist's private values and judgments into the ethics of compulsory treatment of a non-volitional patient. Aspects of this problem are: the safeguarding of human rights during mental illness; the extent of the responsibility to be assumed for the mentally sick person; the problem of the patient's consent; the use of confidential information about the non-volitional patient; and the length to which the therapist may go to attain his ends. Psychosurgery is a particular case in point.

How far may a patient be encouraged to adopt courses of behaviour forbidden or disapproved in his religion but believed to be in the interests of mental health? This situation may not arise as often as is sometimes claimed; but with a proper understanding between patient and therapist the area of serious misunderstanding may be narrowed.

A division of labour between mental health worker and minister of religion, though essential, is not an adequate substitute for a proper understanding by the mental health worker of the culture and religions of the people and, on the part of the minister of religion, a comparable familiarity with principles of mental health. In working out details of the co-operation between mental health workers and ministers of religion, it is necessary to allow for a high degree of specialization of mental health workers' skills, but it is also important that science does not become the sole value of the mental health worker. In less sophisticated societies mental health workers should build up their practice gradually, in harmony and understanding with the community and not in competition with other healing institutions. There is a world-wide shortage of personnel with full training and skills and it is very important to make every use of personnel already in the field.

A number of specific situations encountered in mental health work are discussed. These include the rigidity of the Brahminical system; the possibility of religious actions (e.g. vows) being misinterpreted as mental illness; the difficulties of the student (often quite a young girl) who has suddenly emerged from a protected place in her own society into university life in a foreign culture;

and the troubles caused when the education received by the student abroad conflicts with religious and tribal observances at home. A specific difficulty faces mental health work in some countries where boys are valued more highly than girls.

The discussion extends into the more theoretical area of considering possibilities of difference in intensity of relationship deriving from different family forms. It is important to consider the style of family organization in planning mental health strategy. A special situation exists in the case of a society that is exposed to change by force of events, against its will.

The nature and interrelationship of intuition, objectivity, sympathy, and rapport are briefly discussed.

CHAPTER 4

Some Leads into Research

IT HAS been repeatedly remarked in the foregoing discussion that more exact knowledge is needed, that research and inquiries should be started in many directions in the field of mental health. However, there are several different conceptions in existence about the nature of scientific research in the field of human endeavour.

Research is a great modern talisman and in respect of the physical sciences has reached a level of mathematical precision mainly by the use of techniques of controlled observation and experimentation. For success, research in the physical sciences has depended upon the successful isolation of factors, as required for purposes of control and for narrowing the experimental field.

In the field of biology the application of strict mathematical methodology can be very difficult indeed, especially in relation to the provision of controls and the limitation of variable factors. However, a great deal of methodological progress has been made in biological research generally. In the particular field of human behaviour, much methodological progress has been made in the investigation of the broadest sociological phenomena and in the interpretation of mass statistics. Anthropological studies have made progress making use of what might be termed historical experiment, studying the unfolding of historical events. In the field of microsociological studies less progress has been made, especially in attempts that have been made to construct experimental situations that are comparable with those used in the physical sciences. However, even here progress has been made by the use of new methods of analysis.

The problems in the field of research into interpersonal and small group relations are most complex, and nowhere more so than in respect of human attitudes. The mere isolation and identification of variable factors is often impossible, to say nothing of their limitation and control. Perhaps most difficult of all is the provision of control groups which rarely, if ever, enable experiments to be conducted with the validity now demanded in natural-science research.

Obviously, controlled experiment or observation can be undertaken only in very exceptional circumstances such as, occasionally, in times of war or national emergency when an experimental situation may be set up by circumstances. The observational studies made on young children separated from their mothers in wartime provided an example of the gaining of knowledge from such an historically determined experimental situation.

It appears to us that in respect of the subject of attitudes in various religions and their relationships to concepts of mental health, the next step needs to be the general one of the formulation of schemes of observation and description, by methods that are broadly comparable. It is to be hoped that, by the careful description of phenomena, progress will be made in the identification of problem areas; that is, the definition of problems that appear to offer some prospect of solution by the limited means to hand. With this modest and limited aim in view, this chapter has been entitled 'Some Leads into Research'.

It is proposed first to give some leads into research which have been suggested more specifically in the course of the discussions on mental health and value systems. In each case the first step is to identify the problem area, survey the problem more closely, and investigate how appropriate inquiries might fruitfully be made. The next step would then be to construct working hypotheses.

This chapter is divided into four sections: first, human developmental processes; second, various psychological mechanisms in relation to religion; third, some important mental health practices, and the roles and functions of mental health workers; and fourth, some leads into research of a more general nature, suggested by but not necessarily restricted to the current study of mental health and value systems.

A further preliminary note of warning should be sounded, that any process of inquiry will engender attitudes among the people in the sample under investigation towards the experience of being studied. This inevitable complication of studies of human behaviour will, if not properly allowed for, have a serious distorting effect on the investigation.

On the one hand, the attempt is sometimes made to study individual or group behaviour without the knowledge and consent of the persons who are under observation. Not only is it very difficult to study people without their knowledge, but also, in the opinion of many people, the attempt to do so is ethically undesirable. Some workers regard concealed observation as scientifically unreliable because of the strains and insecurity of an attempt to conceal the situation from the group under observation. On the other hand, the problem in the case of open observation of individual and small group behaviour is that of the effect of the presence of observers. This can produce distortions not only by conscious participation in or resistance to the observation process, but also by unconscious reactions of the subjects.

These problems of subject and observer interaction constitute the first major technical obstacle which needs to be studied and overcome.

HUMAN DEVELOPMENT

Processes by which the Child Becomes Oriented

It is possible that a number of universal phenomena may be found in the area of the establishment in the child of intuition, of empathy, and of unanalysed areas of cognitive understanding. However, the actual forms which such developments will take are almost certainly deeply affected by cultural influences, such as have been discussed. Comparative studies in selected cultures might throw light on the processes by which the child orients himself in his material environment and then relates this orientation to his human emotional environment. It should not be difficult to identify cultures in which the processes of material orientation differ according to cultural patterns (p. 173).

Development of the Child's Systems of Communication

Arising out of the preceding is a field of investigation into the systems of communication which exist between individuals and environment in given cultures, in both their emotional and their cognitive aspects. It may be cited as a hypothesis that it is important for mental health that these systems of communication work well and smoothly.

On page 205 we have considered a speculation that the development of intuition in a child may be a factor of the system of communication that is established between the child and his material and human environment. Out of this speculation a plan might be made to investigate these questions in a number of selected cultures. A working hypothesis could be suggested that the system of communication that is characteristic of a culture will vary according to the pattern of organization of experience and of unconscious interpersonal responsiveness (which may be akin to intuition) that has been established. The precise field of study intended is that of the actual physical and moral training experiences that the toddler child has; his stimulations and restrictions, rewards and punishments, and the manner in which these are conveyed to him, and so on. It is possible that the learning patterns of the child in these respects will have different signficance in various social classes, and varying time relationships in different social classes and societies. These differences will add the variable of the child's development to the existing variables of parental attitudes and behaviour, as determined by many cultural factors. It is likely that different combinations of these variable factors can lead to many possible types of organization of communications.

Differing Patterns in Family Life

We have referred to a number of different patterns in the style of family living and have raised the question of the relationships of these to concepts of mental health (pp. 105, 140-7). The fol-

lowing research areas are of practical importance: (i) comparative studies of the effects of child-mother separations at certain
ages of the child, in cultures which have different degrees of
intimate association of mothers and children, and also in which
standard maternal attitudes may show differences; (ii) comparative studies of the processes by which the new generation takes
over responsibility from its predecessors. Among the questions to
be investigated would be the nature of the hierarchy of authority
if one be present; the social devices to deal with sibling pressures
and rivalries; what happens to the father-figure in a sibling-
oriented society (pp. 146–7); social attitudes towards the father-
figure when the latter has ceased to carry authority, as, for
example, extermination at one extreme to retention as a benevo-
lent influence or some intermediate outcome.

Interruption of Mother-Child Relationships

A related, though at present theoretical, question is that of the
intensity of interpersonal human relationships in a given society
(pp. 200–03). The quality of intensity may have an important
bearing on family and social organization and on attitudes and
behaviour of people under conditions of change (see also p. 231).

More explicit, an inquiry might be made into the effects of
interruption of the maternal-child relationship at given ages in
early infancy in cultures broadly representative of a nuclear type
of family organization and an extended-type family organization,
respectively. Making due allowance for any differences that could
be ascribed to the likely absence of mother-substitutes in the
nuclear-family situation, the inquiry would be directed at differing reactions not only to maternal separation but also to other
forms of change. Parallel studies of children's character formation
in relation to comparable family systems could be planned, also
taking into account the factors arising out of attitudes determined by the prevailing religion and differing cultural patterns
within a common religion.

Definiteness of Conviction

It is possible that the quality or degree of intensity of interpersonal relationships may have some connection with definiteness of conviction, whether religious or other (p. 139). This might be studied in the case of two religions, or preferably two branches of the same religion, one with precisely defined convictions and the other with a generally less definite or undefined religious position. The chief interest would be in the manifestations of individual anxiety in the society concerned. Also the exposure of individuals to alternatives of choice might have some relation to form of social patterns.

'Productive Disintegration'

On pages 107–11 there is some discussion of a state of dynamic equilibrium between constancy on the one hand and differentiation on the other. The existence of regulating mechanisms was postulated (p. 115) to maintain the balance between participation in the outer world and the psychic work that is performed on experiential material. It is suggested that, in the course of development from one phase to another, the existing order will disintegrate and that sometimes such disintegration is seen only as a breakdown of an established order and not as the beginnings of a new phase.

Studies of children's behaviour might be made at various critical phases of development, such as weaning, going to school, and during adolescence, with a view to differentiation between patterns of breakdown of established habitual behaviour that represent essential disintegration and those that form an interim phase in a new constructive advance.

The Constructive Use of Adolescence

An important field of study of great social significance is the extent to which the specific developments of puberty and adolescence are used constructively for religious development and general social good. The phenomena of difficult and antisocial adolescent behaviour is common to all urbanized and changing cultures. This wide field of potential study ranges from the phenomena of the 'beat' generation in the U.S.A. and its analogues in other countries to student behaviour, including political unrest, in many countries.

Inability to Regress, and Rigidity

Another related topic concerned with 'productive disintegration' of adolescence and other periods is the occurrence in some groups of an inability to regress, as shown by intolerant and rigid behaviour in the face of the threat of the loss of established and habitual ways of life. A variant of this, it may be, is the type of conventional organization as seen in a secret society that is resisting social evolution, for example, the Ku Klux Klan or the Mafia, groups that have an extraordinary resistance to change, particularly changes in social attitudes. A third variant of this which is worth study is a degree of apathy towards the future that is sometimes seen among adolescents who are anxious about growing up; an apathy and lack of interest which is a constant source of difficulty to youth-club workers and others attempting to catch the interest of young people. Adaptive behaviour toward mental illness might also come into this field of study (p. 110).

STUDIES IN PSYCHOLOGY AND RELIGION

Studies of Character Formation by Culture in a Common Religion

In the case of a common religion that has spread across cultural boundaries, it might be possible to select and compare two differing cultures which have a religion that is common in its essentials. At a later stage, studies of the differences which national characteristics may make to the religions themselves, as for example the differences in Buddhism as practised in Burma, Thailand, and Japan, might be added.

Definiteness of Social Role

The discussion on pages 143–5 open a wide field for possible investigation into the relationship between definiteness of social role, social mobility, and anxiety.

Parental Priestly Role

The field of study suggested in the preceding paragraph could include, among other subjects, studies of parental status in different religions and cultures. There is also a related question of the effects on family life and child development where the head of the family has a priestly role to fulfil as part or all of his normal social function. This situation might be compared, by religion and culture, with the effects on family life and child development in families in which the head of the family is a priest by virtue of an assumed vocation.

Psychological Treatment and Parental Role

Another aspect of studies of parental status is the effect that therapy for psychological difficulties may have on parent-child relationships. In those cases in which the parent is the patient, some effect may be anticipated upon the style of parental functioning. When the offspring is the patient it would be reasonable to anticipate changes in the offspring's existing relationship with parental authority. It is possible that such changes may be an important issue in cases where parental authority has been strong and in which it may conflict with treatment and itself be affected or possibly destroyed in the process.

Individual Aspirations and Community Goals

We have discussed the questions of how far aspirations involving change may be possible in a given culture, and what levels of response at an aspiration level will be found among various classes of individual in a given society (pp. 75, 87, 125–30).

One aspect of this question (p. 87) is the effect on individual mental health of the strains imposed by responding to environmental demands. A specific instance would be the stimulation of certain desires in an indivdual by a society that did not permit of their satisfaction. It appears to be a valid generalization that all great religions provide aspirations up to which the community may look. The questions to study are to what extent is it open to and possible for the ordinary individual to perceive the aspirational goals of the religion of his community and to move towards them? There may be a great variation between the principles of the religion and the level, in practice, of the goals of aspiration open to the ordinary person, as for example, in the case of the lower-caste Hindus, among whom it is not practically possible for individuals to attain the level of abstract denial of life that the principle of Nirvana demands.

Another interesting possibility for study is the effect, in some societies of a loss of what might be termed elevated goals, a blurring of the focus of aspiration; or, in practical terms, the aim of securing lesser goods for the greatest possible number rather than more highly abstract aims necessarily restricted to very few. Take for example, a problem that is obvious to the people concerned, about which they conceive that something must be done, e.g. psychotic behaviour. A trans-cultural study of treatment aspirations might be effected in this field, to inquire into what people actually do in such a problem in relation to the nature of the community goals and values.

'Maturity at Age' and Religious Ideology

The concept of 'maturity at age' has been introduced as a possible indicator of mental health in childhood (p. 75). This notion compares an all-round assessment of the child's development – physical, intellectual, emotional, and social – with the expectations of society in respect of children of the same age and sex. Though complicated, there seems to be no technical reason why rating-scales should not be developed in these respects. It might then be valuable to undertake studies of children's attitudes to the religious ideology of the culture, in such matters as their readiness and capacity to accept the religious teaching that is normally given.

Of particular importance, it is suggested, is the quality of the child's early relationship with its environment. Satisfaction in early experiences is more likely to lead the child to identify positively with, and therefore to be more receptive to, religious teaching – a hypothesis that appears to be capable of being tested.

Efficacy of Religious and Ethical Instruction

It is a short step to inquiring into the efficacy of religious and ethical instruction at different age levels: first, the type and quality of instruction that is given; and second, the receptivity of the individual to such instruction and experience at different age levels. We would suggest a practical approach from two negative angles: first, the possible harmful effects resulting from instruction when the child is not mature enough for the level at which the instruction is given; and second, the possible destructive effects of instruction at a given age level in cases of individual vulnerability.

A hypothesis could be advanced: that highly emotional teaching before puberty is likely to be ineffective in the long run; during adolescence it may be destructively disturbing; that highly intellectual teaching before puberty will tend to bore children and persuade them that religion is both incomprehensible and dull; i.e. that instruction that is too intellectual before puberty and too emotional at adolescence may be destructive in both cases.

Compulsive Ritualism

Under the heading of compulsive ritualism we would advance four fields of religious and psychological phenomena for study. First, is a study of compulsive and mechanical rituals of prayer in relation to the kind of religion in which they exist: in what circumstances they are encouraged and form part of the normal behaviour pattern of the religious person; where they are accepted but not encouraged; where they exist in special circumstances; and where they are discouraged or forbidden. The specific mental health interest is the relationship between compulsive trends in the individual and the development of ritual practices in his religion.

Second, an investigation might be made into the persistence of archaic and pregenital fantasy constructs, such as magical power and placation ceremonies in ritual, and the degree of overtness which obtains there.

Third, a study might be made of the concreteness of religious

Mental Health and Value Systems

symbolism and its relationship to the psychological needs and reactions of the individual. For example, there is a wide variation within Christianity in the use made of the concept of the blood sacrifice: at one end of the scale human sacrifice has been known, such as the practice of the Mexican penitents who enacted a crucifixion each year; at the other extreme, highly abstract doctrines of atonement, and so on, can be found among sects in which symbolical ritual is taboo. A fourth area could be that of asceticism and its significance in respect of the individual, e.g. comparing popular attitudes and psychiatric attitudes to ascetic behaviour.

Ritual Practices and their Analogies in Compulsive Behaviour

There is a related area of study in the mental health of the individual in relation to prayer practices as they exist in various religions; particularly in comparison with other practices that lead towards the isolation of the individual, in contemplation, and so on. Such practices include, on the one hand, techniques of concentration and relaxation, Yoga and fasting practices; and, on the other, ecstatic dances, gyration, and so on.

Neurosis and Psychosis among Religious People

It is frequently stated that neurosis is more prevalent among religious people than among non-religious people, though, as far as we are aware, this is no more than an expression of an opinion that is commonly prejudiced against religion and is not supported by the evidence of any reliable investigations. While it does not seem practicable at present to embark on direct studies of the relationship between religious feeling and neuroticism, it might be rewarding to undertake some studies of the religious attributes of neurotic patients, in various religions, and also in differing cultures within a common religion.

An hypothesis worth investigation is that there are certain vulnerable positions in society which impel people towards religion or, in other circumstances, into neurosis, e.g. the position of the poorly educated person in a society dominated by the middle class.

Some Leads into Research

There appears to be a widespread tendency among people to associate psychosis with some sort of religious visitation, as indicated by the prevalence, which we have noted, of demoniacal concepts of mental illness and the many differing attitudes to such phenomena as ecstasy. More specific investigation of these problems is essential for better understanding.

We would advocate, also, an increase in the research attention to the underlying personality formation of those who later develop remote or psychotic trends in their religious life.

There are other psychodynamic mechanisms of a more or less pathological nature that have to do with people's beliefs and about which not enough is known. Extensive research conducted in the United States during the late 1940's into the Authoritarian Personality (see Adorno, *et al.*, 1950) pointed to the conclusion that psychopathological processes tended to occur relatively more often among those who had rigid and intolerant viewpoints.

The Selection of Personnel of Religious Missions

A specific question of interest to all propagating religions is that of neurosis among missionaries. It is often stated, though without factual backing, that Christian missionaries are very prone to neurosis. There are certain circumstances of isolation and of frustration of single-minded aims that make this not impossible; and there appears to be justification for a considerable augmentation of several current attempts to make a psychological assessment of intending missionaries. Another study of importance is of the danger signals and warning signs of excessive strain upon individuals (see p. 104).

(see p. 104)

MENTAL HEALTH PRACTICES

Different Ways of Introducing Mental Health Work

On pages 200-8 we have discussed a number of theoretical points relating to the intensity of the child's relationship with the mother and have introduced the notion of a 'built-in' attitude of satisfaction in change. The question was raised there of the possibility of devising different types of approach for newly undertaken mental health work in a parent-oriented society and a sibling-oriented society, respectively.

There is a wide field for investigation represented by the types of mental health approach that are most appropriate to various societies, according to their different forms of organization. The inquiry could be linked with other inquiries into the question of the introduction of change to human societies; in particular to societies that include different religions, or divisions within a common religion.

It would be interesting to investigate the hypothesis that in a nuclear-family society, change tends to emerge spontaneously from within and to be carried forward by the momentum of the satisfaction that individuals find in changing; that such a society tends to resist change that is identified with an alien origin. Conversely, a stable extended-family society tends to be unproductive of spontaneous change; but in a time of general social change tends to be vulnerable to change introduced from outside, at some risk of a breakdown of the existing order, and ensuing social confusion. This is an oversimplification of an enormous problem area, parts of which appear to be open to study.

A problem of great contemporary importance is that of change forced by circumstances (see p. 203). No part of the modern world can insulate itself from changing circumstances and change in others. Much more attention should be paid to the subject of inevitable change, how tragedies can be avoided, and how the greatest benefits from change can be secured.

Differentiation of Function

There is a field of study of general social interest in the extent to which society differentiates functions, i.e. that designated individuals perform certain functions vicariously for the rest of society. For example, in some societies a small group of people may be deputed, as it were, to be religious on behalf of the whole of society, the remainder being very little concerned with religious responsibility (see p. 219). The question arises as to whether a similar phenomenon occurs in the existence of a small criminal class in an otherwise law-abiding society, and a small group of drug-takers, alcoholics, etc. The mental health interest here would be to study the effects of this specialization of role on the mental health of individuals in the community as a whole; and, conversely, the effect of such specialization of role upon any attempt to introduce change as in new mental health work.

Respect of Patients' Values

Coming now to a more strictly psychiatric topic of study, we would like to see undertaken some studies of the diagnosis and treatment of psychiatric patients who have also a genuine and specific religious concern, as distinct from those who are suffering from more general depressive reactions and guilt feelings of a more or less morbid nature. In principle also this idea might be applied to patients with other 'concerns', e.g. artistic, poetical, or musical (see p. 181).

The Role of the Mental Health Worker in the Absence of Specific Value Systems

The role of the mental health worker in the absence of religion or a specific value system is a subject that deserves study. We have discussed some of the issues involved in a division of labour between the mental health worker and the minister of religion (pp. 188–92). We would advocate that inquiries be made into the case of a patient who has no religion, where the final aim of the mental health worker may be difficult to define. We would suggest that the role of the mental health worker in such conditions is more than to aim to produce health and less than to aim to produce perfection. The role could be epitomized as that of helping people to formulate values of their own choice. It would be of interest to investigate to what extent such aims can be identified among mental health workers.

Mixed Marriages

Differing patterns in family life, such as have been discussed in several places (see pp. 140–7), sometimes gave rise to problems which may cause great difficulties in marriages between people of different cultures or different religious faiths. There is no agreement at present as to whether mixed marriages give a greater or a lesser chance of happiness. No doubt the cultural factors are too complex for a simple criterion of this kind to be applied. One suggestive fact has emerged from time to time in studies of mixed marriages, that they tend to be relatively infertile as compared with homogeneous marriages. It is possible that this fact relates to a number of important psychological issues. A related problem of great complexity is that of the religion of children born to mixed marriages, and it would be important to set up studies in depth of the ways in which these problems are tackled, and the outcome.

Introduction of Children to Concepts of Right and Wrong

On page 147 the question was raised: at what point in the child's development is the difference between right and wrong pointed out, and by whom? This has been related to a distinction that is sometimes made between guilt and shame. The field for investigation here is to what extent in a given culture the child's concepts of right and wrong arise out of its individual identification with the mother-figure at a very early age; or alternatively, to what extent the group structure of the family is involved, as in an extended-family situation (see also p. 96).

Introduction of Children to Knowledge of Suffering and Death

On pages 157–62 there has been some discussion of the possible effect on community attitudes and education of the modern practice, which has been cited in the U.S.A., of protecting children and young adults from experience of death. Investigation might reveal the existence of certain mental health principles concerning the way in which children should be introduced to the fact that living things, including human beings, die. Such principles may vary a great deal according to the style of life of the community concerned.

This inquiry might be extended into the consideration of a number of other universal situations to which children must be exposed at some period during their life, e.g. being left on their own, losing their bearings, etc.

Attitudes towards Mental Illness

Brief discussions can be found on pages 97–101 and 162–4 of varying attitudes towards mental illness. This is an essentially practical though complicated field of inquiry, which is extremely important when any programme for introducing mental health services is involved. On page 99 we have referred to the possible danger, when undertaking psychiatric work in a community for the first time, of invading the sheltered position of the people whom it is intended to help, without doing anything commensurate for them.

We would advocate a programme of investigations in various cultures into the contributions which can be made by eccentric people in their own society as compared with the harm that they may do. Follow-up studies of the employment history of psychiatric patients would be relevant in this connection.

As we have seen, a great part of people's attitudes towards mental illness is a reflection of their conceptualization of mental health, which involves practically the whole substance of the present study. However complicated, it is clearly important in any community where mental health work is in existence to get at the attitude of the ordinary person towards mental illness. At the outset, relatively simple measures would be useful; for example, in a fairly simple society, to collect opinions from key people as to the various behaviour phenomena which they would regard as signifying mental disorder. Having arrived at some consensus on a scale of criteria of mental disorder, the same people could be asked to enumerate the individuals in their district whom they regard as falling within these criteria. The material so obtained in simpler societies might provide a starting place for more sophisticated societies. In more highly developed communities the level of sophistication of such studies would, naturally, have to be raised very considerably; and this is a most complicated issue which is the subject of specific projects of inquiry at the present time.

Growth, Change, and Maturity

On pages 107–9 we have discussed certain aspects of human beings during the course of growth and maturation. The concept of 'Maturity at Age' has been used (pp. 75 and 220) in reference to suggested studies of the effects of religious instruction. In general, not enough is known about individual patterns of development, and a common shortcoming of studies of physical, intellectual, and emotional growth is that the norms in use have been based mainly on cross-sectional studies, and therefore do not reflect individual variations in rate of development, such as early spurts and late developing.

In respect of physical growth, a good deal of progress in techniques of assessment has been made by means of long-term studies including descriptive and biometric methods set against radiological studies of bone development. The establishment, with a good degree of accuracy, of the existence of a standard sequence of bone development, has enabled more reliable information to be gathered about patterns of individual physical growth.

In the field of intellectual development, limited progress has been made in finding more refined techniques of assessment, though it is still generally true that mental test norms are based on cross-sectional studies; so that a great deal of work remains to be done. A further difficulty in making longitudinal studies of intellectual growth has been that of finding a method of assessment which, like the radiological assessment of skeletal growth, does not influence the growth pattern itself.

In respect of emotional and social growth and maturation, the technical difficulties of assessment are very great indeed. However, a considerable number of valuable long-term studies are in progress and it is probable that as these studies mature, during the course of the next few years, our knowledge of these areas of child development will be greatly augmented. It is important that an immediate start be made on parallel, comparative studies in other cultures so that the cross-cultural exchange of knowledge can be increased from its present almost non-existent level. Not the least technical difficulty to be overcome is that the part played by environmental influences in emotional and social development is relatively more complicated than in physical and intellectual development, and cross-cultural studies are much needed to elucidate these matters. More specifically, we would encourage the setting up of studies of concepts of child maturation that can be found in various religions and ideologies, in the field of expectations in respect of children, and community reactions to children's retardation or failure. Conversely, studies of children's developing concepts of the religion or ideology of the social group might give valuable information about emergent attitudes.

The great and often insurmountable difficulty of embarking on these vital long-term studies is the big span of time required. In this field it is a case of planting so that others may reap. Nowhere in the field of biological research is there a greater need to cultivate a long-term attitude. In the present state of knowledge and with careful sampling to provide as much reliable social comparison as possible, much of our present knowledge about sequences of emotional development can be clarified by suitable longitudinal studies, and the way opened for more exact techniques of measurement.

Adaptive Behaviour

On pages 109–10 we have suggested that an individual's capacity for adaptation may lead in the direction of mental ill-health as well as mental health, that, for example, psychotic behaviour is a form of adaptation to intra-psychic processes. There is therefore an important field of study in the differentiation between adaptive behaviour leading towards health and ill-health respectively. We suggest that a hypothesis might be constructed which used the notion of certain forms of regressive behaviour as indicative of unhealthy processes, but it is essential that all interpretations made about behaviour should have due regard to the cultural setting. The success of such investigations, therefore, may depend on the state of knowledge of cultural developmental patterns as discussed in the preceding paragraph.

Identity

An important area for study is the nature of the centre of focus of the individual's identity, or the form which a hierarchy of identities may take (pp. 111 and 131). We have discussed that the key question in this field might be the answer to the question 'Who am I?' and it would be interesting to attempt to relate the answer to style of family organization and to child-rearing practices.

In the last section of 'Identity' (pp. 50–51), we bring together some emerging ideas with immediate practical mental health interest, which bear upon the question in the preceding paragraph. The most important of these is described as the *Principle of Positivism,* e.g. that a boy should be brought up positively to be a boy and not to be something that is not a girl. This has an important connection with prejudice formation. We also advocate investigation of the conditions which enable a child to grow up and settle down, as it were, in his own identity. The hypothesis is advanced that capacity to change might be related to the smoothness and unbroken nature of the child's development pattern. The concept of belonging is implicit in much of this discussion and its particular relevance to our present study, in addition to that of prejudice, is in connection with leadership, initiation and ordination ceremonies and, at a more abstract level, with the question of a hierarchy of identities.

On pages 131–40 some discussion will be found on identity and flexibility. Many religions propound a belief in immortality, a life after death, and, in some, reincarnation is an important issue. Questions which might be asked here are, what effect does a belief in immortality or in reincarnation, respectively, have upon the concepts of identity that are held in the society concerned? This study would involve not only the concepts of identity that are held but also the order of moral responsibility assumed by the individual.

The point of investigation here is the existence or not of differences, in terms of identity concepts and moral responsibility, between a society in which it is believed that life is a single progression through this world and a society in which it is believed that life is a succession of reappearances in this world. In the former it will be believed that according to the deeds of the individual, so will he be judged and treated in immortality; and in the latter that future recincarnations are largely determined by past conduct. Set against this might be studies of corresponding attitudes in a society in which there is no concept of a transcendental moral judgment, and again, a society in which there is no belief in an after-life. Related subjects in this field of study are questions of differences made in conduct and moral standards by a belief in predestination as compared with a belief in free will; and by a system of individual responsibility as compared with collective responsibility.

Intensity of Emotional Relationships

It has long been recognized that the type of family organization and the relationships that exist within the family will strongly influence the quality of the interpersonal relationships that the children will form. This may have its cultural significance, in that family life within a particular cultural pattern may have a characteristic flavour, as it were, as revealed in such phenomena as autonomy or, conversely, depedence of children, capacity to adapt to change, and so on.

On pages 200–3 a tentative concept of intensity of emotional relationships has been introduced. We would like to see this theoretical formulation followed up by investigations of the qualities of interpersonal relationships that exist within various styles of family organization. A start might be made by comparing the parent-child relationship in a family in which the child has an intimate connection with not more than two adults, with the relationship values in a family in which the child is in the care of perhaps four or five adults, without a dominant attachment to one individual. The investigation could be directed towards the effects of the introduction of change to children by adults, particularly in the important training experiences of the period of life, roughly, between six and thirty months of age.

Mental Health and Value Systems

Flexibility and Tolerance

In the course of discussion we have related questions of change and 'Productive Disintegration' (p. 217) to flexibility and tolerance of change (p. 111). The studies suggested above in relation to intensity of emotional relationships might serve also to throw light on flexibility and tolerance of change. The key phenomena for study here appear to be those processes by which the unmodified primary drives of children become harmonized with affective values; in other words, how the children's ego-centred drives become modified, and to what degree children will come to find satisfaction in reaching the modified goals of the drives. Further areas of study are: the attitude of society to the processes of instinct modification which all small children go through, and how the child's development is related to the concept of maturity that prevails in that society.

Dependence and Independence

A similar topic for investigation is the important subject of the child's progression from total infantile dependence to the position of relative independence that characterizes the adult (pp. 132–140). This question, together with the related question of authority, was widely discussed at some of the earlier meetings leading up to this report, but it has tended to become absorbed at various points in the development of the argument. At the New York conference, to which references have been made, a number of so-called 'dichotomies' were discussed. The 'divergent principles', as we have also termed them, might more properly be regarded as phenomena that have some of the characteristics of contrasts but which might, possibly, also be at opposite ends of a single scale. The first was autonomy as compared with dependence. It would be interesting to investigate the hypothesis that there is a continuous range of human behaviour from the total dependence of the infant, on the one hand, to a very high degree of individual independence, on the other. The specific problem for investigation would be the relationship between childhood training experiences together with the accompanying

attitudes of society, and the range occupied by the culture concerned on a hypothetical dependence-independence scale.

Responsibility

The broad question of responsibility, to which a number of
references have been made (pp. 96, 125–30), has its roots in
most of our areas of discussion. We would advocate study, in
various cultures, of how responsibility is exercised there, both in
regard to the family and to the community as a whole; and the
making of comparable studies of the way in which the individual
child is expected to attain autonomy, and the degree of autonomy
that is required. These studies would need to be related to the
class structure of the society concerned, and to the prevailing
forms of religion, in association with the patterns of family
organization. Similar studies would be valuable in respect of
religious learning by children. A specific suggestion made on
page 96 is that inquiries should be made into the cross-cultural
importance of the attitude that there must be a rational decision-
making aspect of every act for which an individual can be held
responsible and for which he can be condemned. Such inquiries
need to be related also to the degree, in the cultures concerned,
to which the individual or the society is held to be responsible.

Authority

The second of the divergent principles discussed at the New York
meeting, was understanding by the individual, as compared with
the unquestioning acceptance of authority. The suggested field of
study here would be, specifically, the social attitude towards
autonomy and dependence and, more precisely, the values set on
both of these and the ages at which children are required to
conform to certain particular attitudes (see p. 216).

A major mental health interest in this study would be in the
case of psychiatric treatment, when the attitude of the psychiatrist might come into conflict with the patient's social mores. For
example, the treatment aims of a psychiatrist who came himself
from a culture in which autonomy was valued highly might
cause a problem in relation to a patient in a culture where

Mental Health and Value Systems

autonomy was not valued, and vice versa. Another example is in the difficulties which might arise when a psychiatrist was thought by the social group to be undermining parental authority by his treatment; or, on the contrary, as perpetuating the patient in a state of dependence deemed unhealthy by the social group.

Concern for Others

In this next field the question may be epitomized as the comparison of the attitudes prevailing in a religion that includes the neighbour with a religion that does not. Existing differences can be illustrated by comparing the position of traditional Burmese Buddhism, in which the individual is responsible solely for his own soul, with an attitude that is widespread among Christians, of the individual's responsibility for other people. This subject is of particular importance in the modern world in which, for example, circumstances will on occasion make social groups take responsibility for the children of their enemies, even if they have themselves destroyed their enemies.

In the heart of this subject there is the concept of the brotherhood of Man, to which a lot of homage is paid throughout the world today. It would be important to study this concept comparatively, in relation to father- and sibling-oriented societies, respectively.

Individual Involvement in Religious Practice

On pages 77 and 108 the question has been raised of how far a religion or ideology is meaningful to the individual. The centre of this study would be the involvement of the individual member of society in the prevailing religion or ideology. It is possible to conceive of two antithetical situations; in one case the religion of the community is an outward cultural form that serves as a framework; the religious exercises of the community may be delegated to a professional group set aside for this purpose. The general population may subscribe merely to a code of behaviour involving no affective attachment, apart from the general orientation to the values of the society. The other pole is that of the

234

personal involvement of each individual in a religious responsibility for himself, with the possibility of responsibility for others as well. It would be valuable to make comparative studies, of this order, of prevailing attitudes in differing societies; and to study also the introduction of children to responsibilities, when such exist, in each community, respectively.

Levels of Aspiration in a Culture

On page 108 also, the related question is raised of the ethical aspirations of society and its ways of dealing with guilt, sin, shame, etc. It has been suggested that the key question here is, 'What level of aspiration will be expected of the individual?'

The hypothesis might be advanced that, in a culture in which religion was no more than an outward form involving the individual merely in a code of behaviour, the level of aspiration might be low. In this case, it may be possible for a mentally ill person, for example, to adapt to cultural behaviour at a low level of functioning in spite of being seriously deranged mentally. To be more concrete, a person could be catatonic, seriously out of touch and disordered, but provided he did not create any disturbances or offend against public codes of behaviour, and provided there was someone available to provide food and shelter, no visible problem might occur. In contrast would be the society in which a high degree of personal responsibility and involvement in the prevailing ethical and religious ideology is demanded. In such a society, the behaviour of a catatonic individual might be assessed in terms of duty to the community, and so on. He might not be permitted to behave at a low level of cultural adaptation because this would not satisfy the aspirations of the community, and he would be regarded as being in need of treatment.

It would be valuable to go farther than these two illustrations of specific problems, and to study in differing societies the questions of the types of aspiration that are stimulated by society, and the degrees of satisfaction that are allowed within that society (see pp. 77, 87 and 108). These are broad subjects and in practice would probably need to be approached from the

Mental Health and Value Systems

narrower point of view of the study of phenomena connected with feelings of guilt, sin and shame, and duty.

Mental Health and the Goodness or Badness of Man's Nature

We have referred several times to a quite fundamental difference in attitude which may be found as to whether man's nature is essentially good or bad, and as to the possibility of effecting changes in man in one or other direction. This is a wide question of an abstract nature, and it may be possible to devise methods of studying the effects of dominating convictions in one or other direction upon attitudes and values in the mental health field.

Influence of Imagery

On page 124 a suggestion has been made that, if there were a prevailing type of imagery in a population, it might affect the theology and attitude to God of the people. While we recognize that only a minority of people show a dominant form of imagery and that the majority are mixtures in this regard, it does seem possible to identify certain differences of cognitive style, as between cultures, and also a range of expression of art forms, whether visual, auditory, or kinaesthetic, in different directions and with different emphases. There is a potentially rewarding field of study in the attempt to identify such differences where they exist and to relate them to the cultural ideals, the religious attitudes, and the concepts of mental health of the people concerned.

Fanaticism

Finally, it appears to us to be fitting to end with a reference to fanaticism, which is both an age-old and a contemporary problem of quite exceptional importance. Within very recent memory the world has once again been plunged into disaster through fanaticism, and this has been a recurrent experience of humanity throughout history. We would advocate the award of a high priority in mental health research to the study of the psychology of fanaticism. The world urgently needs to understand a great deal more about the nature of the 'true believer' – the person who is certain that there is only one truth, that all other beliefs are false; that there can be only one true answer to every ethical and religious problem and that it is morally culpable to reject this 'truth'. We are here advocating an interdisciplinary, inter-cultural, mental health study of the contemporary position of fanaticism in the world, and of the forms which it is currently **taking.**

EPILOGUE

It is fitting that our inquiry should pursue a full circle and return in the Epilogue to the point of departure in Chapter 1 – viz. the definition of mental health. Our objective, as stated on page 70, has been 'to throw some light on the relationships between concepts of mental health and the notions of religion and ideology'.

Much has been written in the course of the foregoing discussion in support of our view that mental health can never be an entity that can stand on its own, but that it is both a condition or state and a consequence. Mental health, as a state, may be no more than an unfulfilled aspiration, and much of our discussion has been concerned with the nature of the aspirations that need to be fulfilled before mental health can be attained. Mental health, as a consequence, may flow from the fulfilment of the aspirations or at least some approach towards the fulfilment.

We have come to the conclusion that aspirations towards mental health may well be universal, though the capacity to perceive the aspiration and to move towards it will be affected by cultural influences. When mental health work spreads across international boundaries, the question of cross-cultural applicability is likely to become paramount; and it has been our objective in the foregoing pages to illuminate some of the very complex cultural problems that beset the path of cross-cultural mental health work.

It has been repeatedly emphasized that the development of work in the field of mental health requires people with a special knowledge and experience, and that there are only a very limited number of duly qualified people available at the present time. Mental health workers of all types need at least a dual orientation, professionally speaking. They need to have great competence in their chosen professional area: whether this be psychiatry, psychology, social work, anthropology, nursing, or any other relevant discipline. In addition, they need a quality of outlook and experience which might be described as cultural wisdom, which will include an awareness of cultural factors and a knowledge about the particular culture in which they are working. Not the least of their needs is to have an appreciation of the essential contribution to be made by social anthropology and the related sciences of human behaviour. It is not possible to demand that all mental health workers should be fully trained in the cultural field as well as in their own particular profession. Nor can it be required that all workers who enter this field from the side of social and cultural studies should be trained in a mental health discipline, but they need to have an awareness of and a sensitivity to the essentials of the mental health disciplines.

Thus it is necessary for workers in this field, whether they originate from mental health professions or from the social and cultural side, to be competent in both of the main areas of the field, a competence that is greater than that of merely growing up in a particular religion or ideology, or of a general level of experience common to the professional discipline concerned. Unorganized life experience and common sense are not sufficient qualifications.

The historical fact that the modern concept of mental health has originated in the West has resulted in the great majority of workers in the mental health field being drawn from Western industrialized society. The majority are, by origin at least, mainly Christian or Jewish. This is further complicated by the fact that many of the trained members of other cultures in this field themselves come from a Westernized background or have been educated under Western auspices. These facts serve to emphasize the extreme importance of finding the right people in every culture where they can be employed, and training them for their special role in such a way that it does not involve cultural strain and distortion of attitude.

At the moment a totally disproportionate burden is being put on people from areas other than those of Western Christianity and Judaism who are already competent in the mental health field. In training mental health personnel coming from other religions and cultures, a great deal of consideration needs to be given to the period and scope of the study which they will undertake. For an optimal effect it is likely that the period of study needs to be long, and that time has to be given for an acclimatization of attitudes as well as an assimilation of new knowledge. It is certainly not sufficient in this field to take an individual out of his culture, send him for training across the world to a distant country, and expect him then to return fully prepared as a mental health worker in his own country. There is no more important problem in the international mental health field than the training of personnel for work in places that are freshly being opened up to mental health work.

REFERENCES

ADORNO, T. W., FRENKEL-BRUNSWIK, ELSE, LEVINSON, D. J., SANFORD, R. N. (1950). *The authoritarian personality.* New York: Harper.

ALEXANDER, F. (1931). Buddhist training as an artificial catatonia. *Psychoanal. Rev.* **18**, 129–145.

ALEXANDER, F., & ROSS, HELEN (Eds.) (1952). *Dynamic psychiatry.* Chapter by Margaret Mead. Chicago: University of Chicago Press.

BATESON, G., & MEAD, MARGARET (1942). *Balinese character: a photographic analysis.* New York: Academy of Sciences special publication.

BELO, J. (1960). *Trance in Bali.* New York: Columbia University Press.

BOWLBY, J. (1951). *Maternal care and mental health.* Geneva: WHO; London: H.M.S.O.; New York: Columbia University Press. Abridged version, *Child care and the growth of love.* Harmondsworth: Pelican Books, A. 271.1953.

CLARK, K. B. (1955). *Prejudice and your child.* Boston: Beacon Press.

ERIKSON, ERIK (1950). *Childhood and society.* New York: Norton.

GORER, G. (1959). Pride, shame and guilt: notes on a Montenegrin memoir. *Encounter,* No. 67, April, 28–34.

LOWIE, R. H. (1935). *The Crow Indians.* New York: Farrar & Rinehart.

MEAD, MARGARET (1950). Some anthropological considerations concerning guilt. In Reymert, Martin L., *Feelings and emotions: the Mooseheart symposium*. New York: McGraw-Hill (pp. 362–373).

MEAD, MARGARET (Ed.) (1955). *Cultural patterns and technical change*. UNESCO.

RIESMAN, D., DENNY, REVEL, & GLAZER, N. (1950). *The lonely crowd*. New Haven: Yale University Press.

RÜMKE, H. C. (1953a). *Nieuwe Studies en voordrachten over Psychiatrie*. Scheltema en Holkema, Amsterdam.

RÜMKE, H. C. (1953b). *Problems in the field of neurosis and psychotherapy*. Copenhagen: Munksgärd.

RÜMKE, H. C. (1954). *Mental health in public affairs*. A report of the Fifth International Congress on Mental Health. Solved and unsolved problems in mental health (p. 157). University of Toronto Press.

SIWEK, PAUL (1953). *The riddle of Konnersreuth*. New York: Bruce.

SODDY, K. (1950). *International Health Bulletin* of the League of Red Cross Societies, **2**, No. 2. Mental health.

SODDY, K. (Ed.) (1955). *Mental health and infant development*. London: Routledge & Kegan Paul.

TSUNG-YI LIN (1960). *Reality and vision*. A report of the first Asian seminar on mental health and family life. Manila Bureau of Printing.

WINNICOTT, D. W. (1957). What do we mean by a normal child? In *The child and the family*. London: Tavistock Publications; New York: Basic Books, under title *Mother and child*.

Résumé

CHAPITRE I

EN essayant de définir la santé mentale, l'on tend de plus en plus à mettre l'accent sur les facteurs 'positifs'. Les théories courantes se préoccupent de l'équilibre interne de l'individu, de la qualité des rapports entre l'individu et autrui, et de l'attitude des groupes envers ces rapports.

La discussion porte sur plusieurs questions ; par exemple, le concept de la santé mentale et le comportement qui en dérive, ont-ils la même signification pour tout le monde? Quel est le rapport entre des facteurs tels que l'approbation sociale, le bonheur, le concept du bien, l'adaptabilité, la conformité, la maturité, l'harmonie sociale, le contentement, la croyance en Dieu, etc. et le concept de la santé mentale? L'adaptabilité fournit un exemple utile. Les sociétés acceptent à des degrès différents les variations dans l'adaptation de l'individu. Le rapport entre l'adaptabilité et la santé mentale, est-il influencé par de telles variations? Quelle est la situation au point de vue santé mentale d'un individu s'étant adapté aux valeurs morales particulières d'un culte religieux mineur qui est en désaccord avec la société en général? Si nous admettons que l'adaptabilité est un facteur important dans la santé mentale, est-il possible que l'adaptabilité peut elle-même conduire également à la maladie mentale, comme dans le cas du sujet psychotique qui s'identifie à son processus pathologique? Jusqu'à quel point le manque d'adaptabilité contribue-t-il aux stresses sociaux qui peuvent nuire à la santé mentale.

Un comportement non-conformiste signifie-t-il une santé mentale déficiente? Puisque les attitudes sociales ont tendance a changer, le critère de l'acceptation sociale d'un comportement donné n'est pas valable. Quel est le degré de non-conformisme dans le comportement pour lequel la société rend l'individu responsable ? Presque toutes les sociétés reconnaissent comme irresponsable un certain degré de non-conformisme dans le comportement, mais dans toutes les sociétés nous savons que l'on exigera une responsabilité individuelle en ce qui concerne certaines déviations dans le comportement que l'on juge comme étant moralement inadmissibles.

Jusqu'à quel point les sociétés diffèrent-elles entre elles en ce qui concerne leur tolérance envers les déviations de comportement, et dans quelle mesure tiennent-elles compte des sujets eccentriques et non-conformistes dans la structure même ces sociétés ? Le comportement 'extatique' constitue un domaine où les opinions de la religion et de la psychiatrie se chevauchent et entrent fréquemment en conflit.

Malgré les nombreuses thèses soutenues au sujet des facteurs constituants de la santé mentale, nos connaissances précises sont en fait insuffisantes. Est-il possible de s'aventurer au delà de généralités telles que : les nourrissons ont besoin de l'amour et des soins de leur mère ?

Parmi les questions soulevées relatives au concept de la santé mentale dans la société, nous relevons les suivantes : les valeurs attribuées aux relations affectives entre les membres de la famille sont-elles les mêmes dans toutes les religions ? La santé mentale est-elle compatible avec l'acceptation d'une situation sociale soit inférieure soit supérieure, que ce soit dans le cadre des rapports individuels ou inter-groupes ? De quelle façon les concepts de l'indépendance, de la maturité, etc. varient-elles selon les différents terrains culturels ? Chez le sujet moyen dans la société existe-t-il des variations dans le degré de participation dans la religion ou l'idéologie du groupe, ou dans le niveau d'aspiration exigé de l'individu ? Existe-t-il des sociétés dans lesquelles l'individu peut présenter une adaptation inférieure à la moyenne sans subir de stresses ? Jusqu'à quel point les sociétés ont-elles tendance à promouvoir, permettre ou interdire la satisfaction de tous les désirs provoqués par la participation à une société donnée ?

Dans un sens on peut considérer la santé mentale comme étant un équilibre dynamique entre les facteurs constants d'un côté, et les facteurs de differenciation, de développement et de changement de l'autre.

Toute action entreprise dans le domaine de la santé mentale doit tenir compte des changements qui s'opèrent dans la société en question. Quelle est l'importance dans la santé mentale de la force du moi social, de sa continuité, de sa cohérance et de sa flexibilité ? La conservation de la force du moi social, et par là même de la santé mentale, est-elle possible si des fluctuations dans le comportement, telles que des symptômes psychosomatiques et des phénomènes de dissociation, sont permises sans encourir en période de stress de peines sociales.

Finalement, nous discutons de certaines valeurs universelles relatives à la vie et aux attitudes sociales de l'homme. Par exemple, le développement, qui est un phénomène biologique universel, présuppose la disparition d'un ordre existant et son remplacement par autre chose. Comment peut-on distinguer l'instabilité précurseur d'un nouveau développement de celle qui précède la désintégration ?

CHAPITRE II

Parmi les nombreuses variations que l'on trouve dans les différentes religions et idéologies, on peut distinguer dans le comportement de l'homme un certain nombre de tendances contrastantes. Nous trouvons celles-ci dans une diversité d'associations selon les différentes sociétés. Nous en relevons quelques exemples. Presque partout dans le monde l'on considère les systèmes de valeurs comme étant fixes, mais dans certains cas l'on tient compte du changement et du développement possible (le principe islamique de l'utilité en fournit un exemple).

On considère que l'homme est capable de se perfectionner. Ceci constitue un des principes essentiels du Confucianisme ; les valeurs sont estimées par rapport au rôle et au comportement social, à l'harmonie et au 'juste milieu'. La religion hindoue tient moins compte de la signification morale du comportement social, et considère même que certaines déviations sociales constituent un signe de sainteté.

Beaucoup de religions ont insisté sur le côté non-matérialiste de leurs systèmes de valeurs lesquelles, dans le cas des religions d'inspiration surnaturelle, sont d'ordre transcendant.

Les attitudes envers la responsabilité de l'homme vont de celles qui prétendent que l'homme est naturellement bon et que sa déchéance est due au milieu, jusqu'à celles pour lesquelles l'homme est capable de choisir le mal même dans un milieu social parfait. Le Confucien tient la société responsable du mauvais comportement, mais l'individu est tenu de cultiver le bon qui réside en lui. L'Hindou renvoie la responsabilité à une réincarnation future. Beaucoup de sociétés, parmi lesquelles celle du Nigéria, libèrent la société de toute responsabilité vis-à-vis de l'individu ; et ceci semble s'appliquer de plus en plus à la seconde génération du Marxisme soviétique.

Presque toutes les religions prétendent à un certain degré de flexibilité, mais les concepts varient entre eux. La religion hindoue reconnait une liberté absolue de pensée et subordonne le dogme à l'expérience, mais impose un contrôle sévère du comportement social. La religion hébraique donne une impression de rigidité, mais pratiquée à travers les siècles elle a démontré sa flexibilité remarquable.

La flexibilité peut être erigée en institution, comme dans la philosophie musulmanne du contraversialisme, des 'bénéfices de la pensée floue' et du principe de l'unanimité d'opinion. L'unanimité basée sur le sentiment général donne sa flexibilité à l'Anglicanisme.

Les religions d'inspiration surnaturelle tendent à être flexibles à la fois selon l'époque et selon la distribution géographique, mais dans la plupart des cas il y a une limite à cette flexibilité. Ceci est apparent dans la doctrine catholique selon laquelle les propositions contradictoires ne peuvent être acceptées simultanément et la vérité révélée et formulée en dogme est inflexible. La tolérance vis-à-vis des autres groupes et les variations en ce qui concerne les points non-essentiels ne constituent pas la flexibilité de doctrine.

Un autre aspect de la flexibilité est l'absolu avec lequel se formulent les convictions religieuses. La définition étroite offre

Résumé

à l'individu le choix facile entre appartenance et non-appartenance. Le manque de définition précise peut devenir source d'angoisse pour l'individu.

Quelques exemples sont présentés des différents types d'organisations familiales qui peuvent jouer un rôle dans les études se rapportant à la santé mentale. Les exemples discutés sont : le système familial collectif hindou, avec son large spectre de liens de parenté et la communauté des biens familiaux. Ce système protège les jeunes mais peut également les frustrer. L'organisation familiale confucienne est davantage rigide et le rôle social y est défini de façon explicite. Dans la famille juive on souligne l'amour entre individus, qui détermine le rôle social. Les familles musulmanes considèrent l'autorité comme découlant de la situation privilégiée du père humain auprès de Dieu.

D'importantes distinctions peuvent être établies entre les familles ayant une structure verticale, orientées selon l'autorité paternelle et maternelle, et celles ayant une structure horizontales, frères-soeurs, qui ont tendance à se fragmenter en unités 'nucléaires'.

On constate que le contenu de ce qui constitue le bien et le mal peut varier selon le moment. L'âge auquel on fait comprendre aux enfants la différence entre le bien et le mal est un facteur conceptuel important. D'autres facteurs entrant en jeu sont : les identifications individuelles (la culpabilité) et l'identification collective (la honte). Selon les concepts du bien et du mal, la sexualité peut apparaître sous des angles différents. Pour les Chinois la sexualité apparait essentiellement comme une partie intégrale du rôle parental. Dans la religion chrétienne la sexualité a donné lieu à une forte angoisse et à des polémiques importantes. Ceci est peutêtre dû à la chaude affectivité qui existe dans la famille chrétienne monogamme qui tend à augmenter l'intensité émotive de la sexualité en comparaison avec le mode de vie de la famille polygamme ou collective.

Une nouvelle aspiration peut rendre malsain ce que la société a jusqu'à là jugé comme étant sain. Tout jugement sur la santé mentale des individus doit tenir compte des aspirations qui peuvent exister à l'intérieur du groupe.

Les attitudes envers l'erreur varient également. On peut établir une comparaison intéressante entre la tendance soviétique à la liquidation de l'individu non-conformiste et la politique de récupération courante en Chine communiste. Le travail du psychiatre rencontre souvent des resistances si ses efforts pour guérir l'individu malade sont interprètés comme étant la rédemption d'un individu déviant du comportement social moyen.

Les différentes religions ont des attitudes caractéristiques envers la souffrance et la mort. Dans la religion chrétienne, bien que l'importance de ces concepts varie selon les sectes, l'on trouve à la fois une acceptation positive de la souffrance comme instrument faisant surgir le bien du mal, et la reconnaissance qu'il est le devoir de l'homme de partager la souffrance humaine. La religion confucienne n'accorde pas de valeur positive à la souffrance.

Toute action dans le domaine de la santé mentale doit également tenir compte de l'aspiration universelle 'médicale' qui tend à vouloir soulager la souffrance. Beaucoup de sociétés essayent de protéger les enfants du concept même de la souffrance et de la mort. Par contre, une communauté aux Indes croit que le but essentiel de la vie et de souffrir, et les Hindous, en général, considèrent la mort comme une délivrance des souffrances de ce monde. L'opinion est assez générale qu'un minimum de douleur et de souffrance est nécessaire pour la maturité complète de l'homme.

Dans l'histoire de l'homme les attitudes envers la santé mentale ont été dominées presque universellement par des notions de possession diabolique, qui d'ailleurs existent encore presque partout au monde. D'autres notions ont reçu tour à tour de l'importance : les causes métaphysiques des maladies mentales, les expériences individuelles, les facteurs sociaux et, plus récemment, les facteurs psycho-biologiques.

Dans cette discussion nous ne faisons que schématiser les similarités entre les grandes religions et idéologies. Nous retrouvons au moins quatre courants d'idées communs en ce qui concerne la recherche de la santé : la valeur des efforts intellectuels ; la renonciation de la chair ; la prière afin de com-

248

prendre les mystères ; et la recherche de la santé par l'action. On pourrait également tenir comme général la proposition que l'harmonie entre l'intellect et l'affect, dans le but d'un contrôle intégré du dernier par le premier, favorisera la santé mentale.

CHAPITRE III

Dans le domaine le la santé mentale, un certain nombre d'hypothèses non-prouvées sont couramment acceptées en ce qui concerne la vie de l'individu et de la famille ; par exemple, que le type de vie de famille dans lequel le praticien lui-même a été élevé est 'le meilleur'; que la mère est la personne idéale pour élever son enfant; qu'il y a anthithèse entre les valeurs matérielles et spirituelles. Des hypothèses de diverses sortes sont également acceptées en ce qui concerne la vie contemplative par rapport à la vie active ; au sujet de la sexualité et de la valeur de la procréation ; au sujet du bespoin d'élever le niveau de vie, etc.

Les changements opérés dans le domaine de la santé mentale doivent trouver leur base dans les principes connus de la communauté, en évitant les changements brusque de la structure familiale, telle que l'introduction brusque d'une attitude égalitaire dans une société ayant une structure familiale de type vertical. L'étude de la façon dont les enfants de la communauté sont exposés au changement fournit d'utiles informations. Dans certaines sociétés le changement est un privilège limité à des groupes sociaux restreints, et en d'autres, telle qu'une communauté hindoue orthodoxe, le changement est une éventualité rare ou impossible. Le succès de la promotion de la santé mentale dépend en partie de la création d'un climat favorable au changement et d'un sentiment que le changement est possible et désirable. Dans certaines conditions, les croyances et les traditions établies dans la société peuvent être 'vulnérables' aux idées nouvelles. Beaucoup de pratiques (par exemple, le sacrifice humain, l'esclavage et, jusqu'à un certain point, la polygamie) ne survivent pas dans une société exposée aux valeurs différentes d'autres sociétés. L'amélioration dans la condition de la femme un peu partout dans le monde fournit une bonne occasion pour l'action en faveur de la santé mentale dans les pays où la femme occupe encore une position inférieure.

Ceux qui travaillent dans le domaine de la santé mental doivent avoir une 'compréhension' culturelle mais pas nécessairement une identification culturelle. Comme dans le cas du thérapeute et de ses malades, il peut y avoir des cas où un certain degrè de distance culturelle, qui pourrait n'être qu'une distinction sociale, peut être un avantage. De toute façon, il est nécessaire dans le domaine de la santé mentale de connaître et de respecter les valeurs essentielles de ceux avec lesquels on travaille.

Un partage de la responsabilité entre le thérapeute et le conseiller spirituel est à recommender. La responsabilité en ce qui concerne la vie spirituelle du malade est une question importante dans le rapport affectif médecin/malade. La création d'une empathie dépend en partie du respect témoigné par le thérapeute pour les croyances de ses malades. Si ce respecte existe, l'empathie peut surmonter les divergences religieuses grâce au terrain commun de l'humanité. Menacer les valeurs essentielles d'un individu ou d'une communauté risque d'augmenter le sentiment d'angoisse et d'insécurité.

Il est important de se mettre en garde contre l'introduction inconsciente, dans l'éthique d'un traitement d'office d'un malade non-volontaire, de valeurs et de jugements personnels propre au thérapeute. Nous relevons les aspects suivants de ce problème : la sauvegarde des droits humains au cours d'une maladie mentale, le degré de responsabilité assumé vis-à-vis du malade mental, le problème du consentement du malade, l'usage fait de renseignements confidentiels au sujet du malade non-volontaire, et les moyens que peut se permettre le thérapeute afin d'atteindre son but (la psychochirurgie en est un exemple).

Jusqu'à quel point peut on encourager un malade à adopter une conduite que sa religion interdit ou désapprouve, mais que l'on croit être dans l'intérêt de sa santé mentale ? Cette situation ne se produit pas aussi souvent qu'on le prétend parfois ; mais une bonne compréhension entre malade et thérapeute peut limiter le terrain de mésentente.

Résumé

La division du travail entre le psychiatre et le prêtre, quoiqu'essentielle, ne peut remplacer de façon adequate une véritable compréhension de la culture et des religions de ses malades de la part du psychiatre, et une connaissance comparable des principes de la santé mentale de la part du prêtre. En considérant en détail la coopération entre thérapeute et prêtre, il est nécessaire de tenir compte du haut degré de spécialisation du premier, mais il importe également que la science ne devienne pas son unique point de référence. Dans les sociétés moins évoluées le praticien de santé mentale doit introduire sa spécialité peu à peu, coopérant harmonieusement avec la communauté, et non pas en compétition avec les pratiques 'thérapeutiques' établies. Dans le monde entier on manque de personnel qualifié et il est très important de profiter du personnel déjà actif dans ce domaine.

Notre discussion porte sur un certain nombre de cas particulier rencontrés dans la pratique de la santé mentale. Parmi ceux-ci : la rigidité du système Brahmin ; la fausse interpretation possible des actes religieux (par exemple, des voeux) comme étant des symptômes pathologiques ; les difficultés de l'étudiant (souvent une toute jeune fille) qui, quittant brusquement sa situation protégée dans sa propre société, se trouve projetée dans la vie universitaire d'une culture étrangère ; les problèmes soulevés lorsque l'éducation reçue par l'étudiant à l'étranger entre en conflit avec les pratiques de la religion de sa tribu. On rencontre un problème particulier dans les pays ou les garçons jouissent d'une considération supérieure par rapport aux filles.

La discussion s'étend dans des considérations plus théoriques portant sur les possibilités de différences d'intensité dans les rapports personnels résultant des divers types de structure familiale. Dans l'organisation d'un programme de santé mentale il importe de tenir compte du type de structure familiale. Un cas spécial est celui où une société se trouve exposée aux changements par la force des évènements, et contre son propre gré.

Nous discutons brièvement de la nature de et des correlations entre l'intuition, l'objectivité, la sympathie et le rapport affectif.

Resumen

Las tentativas que se han realizado para definir la salud mental han hecho resaltar paulatinamente factores más "positivos". Las actuales tendencias de enfocar la cuestión se ocupan del equilibrio interno del individuo, el carácter de las relaciones entre el individuo y otras personas, y las actitudes de los grupos sociales hacia dichas relaciones.

La discusión en torno a este tema enfoca diversos factores: por ejemplo, ¿tiene el concepto de la salud mental y su resultante comportamiento diversos significados para diferentes personas? ¿Qué relación existe entre fenómenos tales como la aceptación social, la felicidad, el concepto de la bondad, la adaptabilidad, la conformidad, la madurez, armonía social, la satisfacción, la creencia en Dios, etc., y el concepto de la salud mental? La adaptabilidad constituye un caso tópico. Las distintas sociedades difieren en el grado en que toleran variaciones en la adaptación del individuo. ¿Se halla la relación entre la adaptabilidad y la salud mental afectada por semejantes variaciones? ¿Cuál es la actitud que reviste la salud mental del individuo que se ha adaptado a las características propias de un culto religioso que se halla en contraposición con la sociedad en general? Si se acepta que la adaptabilidad es un factor importante en la salud mental, ¿es acaso posible que la adaptabilidad conduzca también a la enfermedad mental, como ocurre con un individuo atacado de psicosis que se identifica con sus procesos patológicos? ¿Hasta qué punto contribuye la falta de adaptabilidad a provocar tensiones sociales que podrían perjudicar la salud mental?

¿Constituye el comportamiento discordante de una persona un indicio de salud mental precaria? Como quiera que las actitudes sociales tienden a cambiar, el criterio de la aceptación social con respecto al comportamiento no merece confianza. ¿Hasta qué grado del comportamiento discordante hace la sociedad responsable al individuo? Prácticamente todas las culturas admiten que un cierto grado en la perturbación del comportamiento constituye irresponsabilidad, pero sabemos que en todas las sociedades la gente asocia responsabilidad individual en torno a algunos aspectos del comportamiento discordante y lo condenan.

¿Hasta qué punto difieren las sociedades en su tolerancia hacia el comportamiento discordante y aceptan los individuos excéntricos y diferentes en la estructura de la sociedad? El tema del comportamiento estático es un terreno en que ocinciden, y a menudo chocan, las actitudes religiosas y de la "salud mental".

A pesar de las muchas suposiciones que se hacen acerca de los factores constituyentes de la salud mental, el conocimiento exacto en esta esfera resulta insuficiente. ¿Es posible trascender de generalidades tales como "los niños necesitan el amor y el cuidado de sus madres"?

Entre las cuestiones discutidas que conciernen el concepto de la salud mental en la sociedad destacan las siguientes: ¿Es el valor atribuído al afecto entre las personas en el seno de la famila el mismo en el caso de todas las religiones? ¿Es la salud mental compatible con la aceptación de una posición inferior o superior en la sociedad, ya se trate de relaciones entre individuos o grupos sociales? ¿Cómo difieren los conceptos de independencia, madurez, etcétera, en diferentes normas sociales? ¿Existen variaciones en el grado en que la persona corriente da la sociedad se halla comprometida por la religión o ideología del grupo social, o por los niveles de las aspiraciones exigidas del individuo? ¿Existen sociedades en las que los individuos se pueden adaptar a un nivel bajo sin tensiones? ¿Hasta qué punto las sociedades fomentan, permiten o prohiben la satisfacción de todos los deseos que la vida en dicha sociedad estimula?

La salud mental se puede considerar en cierto sentido como un equilibrio dinámico entre la constancia, por una parte, y la diferenciación, el desenvolvimiento y el cambio, por la otra.

El trabajo en torno a la salud mental se debe compaginar

cuidadosamente con el cambio que tiene lugar en la sociedad de que se trata. ¿Hasta qué punto resultan importantes para la salud mental la fuerza de la identidad, su continuidad, coherencia y flexibilidad? ¿Es posible preservar la fuerza de la identidad, y de aquí la salud mental, si se permiten cambios provisionales en el comportamiento, como es por ejemplo la sintomatología psicosomática y los fenómenos de disociación, sin ser objeto de penalidades sociales durante la existencia de tensiones?

Finalmente, se abordan ciertos valores universales relacionados con la vida humana y las diversas actitudes. Por ejemplo, el desarrollo, que es un fenómeno biológico universal, presupone la desaparición del orden existente y su substitución por algo nuevo. ¿Cómo puede distinguirse la inestabilidad que anuncia un nuevo desenvolvimiento del que precede a la desintegración?

CAPITULO II

Entre el gran número de variaciones que ocurren entre las diferentes religiones e ideologías, se pueden identificar varias tendencias contrastantes en el comportamiento humano. Estas se presentan en diversas combinaciones en distintas sociedades. Se discuten algunos ejemplos. En la mayor parte de mundo los sistemas de valores se consideran fijos, pero en algunos casos se admite el cambio y desarrollo (por ejemplo, el principio islámico de la utilidad).

El hombre se considera perfectible. Entre otros, se trata de un importante principio confucionista; y los valores se describen en función de objetivos y comportamientos sociales, armonía y el Medio de Oro. El induismo atribuye menos importancia a la significación moral y el comportamiento social, y considera también a ciertas formas de desviación social como una señal de santidad.

Muchas religiones hacen hincapié sobre los aspectos no materiales de sus sistemas de valores que, en el caso de las religiones de revelación, adquieren una importancia transcendental.

Las actitudes en torno a la responsabilidad humana presentan, por una parte, al Hombre como un producto bueno y malo del ambiente que le rodea, y, por otra parte, al Hombre capaz de optar por el mal incluso en condiciones sociales perfectas. Los confucionistas consideran a la sociedad responsable del comportamiento perverso, pero el individuo teine la obligación de cultivar el bien que hay en su seno. El que profesa la religión del induísmo proyecta la responsabilidad en la reincarnación futura. Muchas sociedades, incluída la de Nigeria, despoja a la sociedad de responsabilidad para el individuo, lo cual se está también evidenciando en la segunda generación del marxismo soviético.

Prácticamente todas las religiones se atribuyen un cierto grado de flexibilidad, pero los conceptos varían. El induísmo permite completa libertad de pensamiento y subordina el dogma a la experiencia pero domina el comportamiento social hasta un grado poco común. La religión hebrea da la impresión de rigidez, pero durante el transcurso de los siglos ha demostrado ser extraordinariamente flexible.

La flexibilidad puede adquirir un carácter institucional, como ocurre en la filosofía musulmana de la controversia, los "frutos de la vaguedad", y el principio del asentimiento. El asentimiento, basado en el sentimiento humano, da flexibilidad al cristianismo anglicano.

Las religiones de revelación tienden a ser flexibles tanto por lo que se refiere al período como, en ciertos casos, a la distribución geofráfica, pero ambos factores imponen un límite a la flexibilidad. Este hecho se evidencia en la insistencia de la religión católica romana de que las proposiciones contradictorias no se pueden aceptar simultáneamente y de que la revelación de la verdad, formulada como dogma, no es flexible. La tolerancia de otros grupos y las variaciones de los elementos no esenciales no son lo mismo que la flexibilidad de la doctrina.

Otro aspecto de la flexibilidad es la exactitud con que se formulan las convicciones. Una estrecha definición ofrece al individuo la simple opción de pertenecer o no. La falta de definición puede producir ansiedad en el individuo.

Se citan unos pocos ejemplos de los diferentes tipos de organización familiar, que pueden afectar el trabajo en torno a la salud mental. Se trata de: el sistema hindú de familia mancomunada con su amplio séquito de parentesco y comunidad. reconocidos por cuanto a la propiedad de la familia. Este sistema protege al joven, aunque también le puede frustrar. La organización familiar confucionista es más rígida y se define explícitamente el objetivo social. En la famila judía, se concentra la atención en el amor entre las personas, que determina la función social. Las familias islámicas consideran que la autoridad proviene de la posición del padre humano, que ostenta la máxima autoridad después de Dios.

Se pueden establecer importantes distinciones entre las familias de una estructura de autoridad vertical, u orientada hacia el padre, y las de orientación estructural horizontal y que tiende a fragmentarse en unidades "nucleares".

A veces se peude descubrir una cierta diferencia en lo que la gente cree, de tiempo en tiempo, como acertado o equivocado. La edad a la que se demuestra a los niños la diferencia entre lo acertado y lo equivocado constituye un importante factor conceptual. Otros factores son, en diferente medida, las identificaciones propias del individuo (culpa) y la identificación colectiva (vergüenza). La sexualidad se presenta principalmente de diferentes modos entre los conceptos sobre lo acertado y lo equivocado. Para los chinos, la sexualidad aparece fundamentalmente como una parte integrante de la función paterna. Los cristianos han revelado gran contrariedad de opinión y ansiedad acerca del tema sexual, lo cual se debe posiblemente al carácter de profundo afecto que impera en la familia monógama cristiana, que ha tendido a aumentar la intensidad emotiva de la sexualidad si se compara con el modo de vida de una familia polígama.

Una nueva aspiración puede convertir en insano la que anteriormente la sociedad consideraba como mentalmente sano. Toda opinión sobre la salud mental de la gente debe tener en cuenta la existencia de las aspiraciones en el seno de dicho grupo.

Las actitudes acerca del error también varían. Se puede

establecer una comparación interesante entre la tendencia soviética a liquidar el individuo divergente y la actual tendencia comunista a redimirle. El trabajo en torno a la salud mental tropieza algunas veces con cierta resistencia si el propósito de curar un individuo mentalmente enfermo se considera como la redención de alguien que se separa del comportamiento socialmente aceptado.

Las diversas religiones adoptan actitudes características hacia el sufrimiento y la muerte. En el seno del cristianismo, aunque se da énfasis a diferentes factores, reviste gran importancia la aceptación positiva del sufrimiento para convertir el mal en bien, y el reconocimiento del deber del Hombre a compartir el sufrimiento de la humanidad. La actitud confucionista niega el valor positivo del sufrimiento.

El trabajo en torno a la salud mental debe también tener en cuenta la aspiración médica universal con miras a impedir el sufrimiento. Muchas sociedades tratan de proteger a los niños contra el conocimiento del dolor y la muerte. Una comunidad india, como contraste, cree que la finalidad principal de la vida es el sufrimiento, y los hindúes, en general, consideran a la muerte como la liberación del sufrimiento en el mundo. Existe el acuerdo relativamente extendido de que para conseguir completamente la madurez humana debe concurrir un cierto elemento de sufrimiento.

Las diversas actitudes acerca de la enfermedad mental durante la historia se han visto casi completamente dominadas por la idea de estar poseídos por el demonio, que todavía prevalecen por casi todo el mundo. Se han observado también tendencias históricas que ponen de manifiesto, en orden sucesivo, las causas metafísicas del desorden mental, las experiencias en la propia vida del individuo, factores sociales y, en años recientes, factores psicobiológicos.

En la discusión se hace únicamente una alusión somera a las similitudes entre las grandes religiones e ideologías. Hay por lo menos cuatro cursos de acuerdo con respecto a la preservación de la salud : el valor del estudio intelectual; la renunciación a las cosas de la carne; devoción para comprender los misterios; y la preservación de la salud por medio de la acción. Tal vez exista acuerdo general en la sugerencia de que la armonía entre la vida cogniscitiva y afectiva, que conduce al dominio integrado por parte de la primera, estimulará la salud mental.

CAPITULO III

Con respecto al trabajo acerca de la salud mental es muy común basarse en suposiciones no probadas sobre la vida del individuo y de la familia; por ejemplo, que el modo de vida familiar en que se educó el practicante propiamente dicho es "la mejor"; que la madre es la persona más indicada para cuidar de su propio hijo; que existe antítesis entre la máquina y los valores espirituales. También se anteponen suposiciones de diversos géneros acerca de la vida activa, en contraste con la vida contemplativa; en lo tocante al aspecto sexual y a la conveniencia de procrear; acerca de la necesidad de elevar el nivel de vida, y así sucesivamente.

Los cambios en la salud mental deben basarse en principios conocidos por la comunidad, debiéndose evitar todo cambio repentino en el sistema familiar, tal como la abrupta introducción en la sociedad de la actitud igualitaria con una estructura familiar orientada hacia el padre. Mucho queda por aprender del estudio en torno a la manera en que los niños de la comunidad quedan expuestos al cambio. En algunas sociedades, el cambio propiamente dicho constituye un privilegio confinado a ciertos grupos sociales exclusivamente, y en otras, como es la sociedad hindú ortodoxa, todo cambio es poco menos que imposible. El éxito en la labor de fomentar la salud mental depende en parte en el establecimiento de un ambiente favorable al cambio y en la creencia de que cambio es deseable y posible.

Las creencias y costumbres establecidas pueden resultar "vulnerables" a las ideas nuevas, bajo ciertas condiciones. Muchas de las prácticas pasadas (por ejemplo, el sacrificio humano, la esclavitud y, hasta cierto punto, la poligamia) no logran sobrevivir en una sociedad que está expuesta a los diferentes valores de otras sociedades. El estado social más avanzado de las mujeres en muchas partes del mundo ofrece una excelente oportunidad para poner en práctica el trabajo de la salud mental en países en donde todavía ocupan una posición inferior.

El practicante especializado en el trabajo de la salud mental debe contar con un entendimiento cultural pero nó necesariamente con una identificación intelectual. Tal y como ocurre en el caso del terapeuta y los pacientes, cuando se trata del especialista en salud mental ye el cliente pueden darse casos en los que un cierto grado de separación intelectual, que tal vez no pase de ser más que una diferencia de clase, resultará ventajosa. En cualesquiera de los casos, el practicante en salud mental debe saber respetar los altos valores de la gente con quien trabaja.

Se aboga por una división de responsabilidad entre el terapeuta y el consejero espiritual. La responsibilidad en la vida espiritual de su paciente es un importante factor en la relación entre el doctor y el paciente. El desarrollo de la facultad de proyectar la propia personalidad en el objeto de contemplación depende, hasta cierto grado, en el respeto que las creencias del paciente merezcan al terapeuta. Con este respeto, dicha facultad puede cubrir amplias diferencias de religión, debido al terreno común de la naturaleza humana. Toda amenaza a los valores centrales de un individuo o de la comunidad aumentan, de modo pernicioso, la ansiedad y la inseguridad.

Es importante impedir la introducción inconsciente de los valores y juicios privados del terapeuta en la ética del tratamiento obligatorio de un paciente no volitivo. Los aspectos que rodean a este problema son: la salvaguardia de los derechos humanos durante la enfermedad mental, el grado de responsabilidad que se asumirá con respcto a la persona mentalmente enferma, el aspecto del consentimiento del paciente, el empleo de información confidencial acerca del paciente no volitivo, y el límite de las medidas que puede tomar el terapeuta para conseguir su propósito. La psicocirujía merece mencionarse por resultar sumamente adecuada.

¿Hasta qué punto se debe estimular a un paciente para que adopte un comportamiento prohibido o condenado por su religión, pero beneficioso para salud mental? Esta situación tal vez no surja con la frecuencia que se alega, pero si existe una comprensión debida entre el paciente y el terapeuta será posible reducir al mínimo las diferencias en pugna.

La división del trabajo entre el practicante en salud mental y el sacerdote, aunque esencial, no constituye el substituto adecuado del entendimiento, por parte del practicante en salud mental, en torno a la cultura y religiones de la gente y, por parte del sacerdote, de un entendimiento comparable de los principios de la salud mental. Al tratar de delinear los pormenores que deben acompañar a la colaboración entre los practicantes en salud mental y los sacerdotes, es preciso aceptar un elevado grado de especialización en la pericia del practicante, pero es tan importante no olvidar que la ciencia no pase a ser el único valor del practicante. En las sociedades no muy sofisticadas, los practicantes en salud mental deben afianzar sus prácticantes gradualmente en armonía y consonancia con la comunidad y nó en competencia con otras instituciones de cura. Existe una escasez mundial de personal con la aptitud y pericia necesarias, por lo que es esencial obtener el mayor provecho posible del personal que actualmente practica.

Se enfocan varias de las situaciones que se presentan durante el trabajo en torno a la salud mental, entre las que figuran la rigidez del sistema Brahmínico; la posibilidad de que ciertos actos religiosos (por ejemplo, los votos) se confundan por enfermedades mentales: las dificultades con que tropieza el estudiante (con frecuencia una muchacha joven) que pasa súbitamente de un lugar protegido en su propia sociedad a la vida universitaria en una cultura extraña; y las dificultades que surgen cuando la educación que ha recibido el estudiante en el extranjero choca con los principios religiosos y tribeños que observa en su país. Otra dificultad importante se da en los países en donde se precia a los varones más que a las hembras.

La discusión pasa luego a la esfera más teórica que consiste en considerar las posibilidades que ofrece la diferencia en intensidad de la relación social en diversas formas de familia. Al planear la estrategia de la salud mental es esencial conocer el tipo de la organización familiar. Se presenta, sin embargo, una situación especial en aquella sociedad que queda forzonsamente expuesta a los acontecimientos, contra su propia voluntad.

Asimismo, se hace una breve alusión a la naturaleza y relación mútua de la intuición, objetividad, simpatía y comunicación.

Index

1. IDENTITY

adolescence, 13
adoption, 44
alcoholism, 16
ancestors, 'remembering', 24–5
Apollo, 49
artificial insemination, 46
Australia, 32

Bali, 34–5
boys, dress of, 33
Buddhism, 34
burial wishes, empathy and, 11–12

child,
    development, 8, 41–2
    maturation, in Israel, 44
child-parent identification, 12–13
Childhood and Society, 36
Chinese, the,
    family, 26
    names and, 22, 28–30
    sons, 25
Chinese Buddhism, 34
'Ching Ming' Festival, 24
Christianity, 23
    in China, 24
'Chung Yeung' Festival, 24
class, 30–1
collectivism, 23–5
Communists, 19
concentration camps, children and,
    19
continuum, 4–5

courtship, 13–14
cremation wishes, empathy and,
    11–12
Czechoslovakia, youth in, 32
culture, identity and, 9, 30–39

Davy Crockett, 40
day-dreaming, 45
death, 26–7
    attitudes to, 49
De Levita, 49
delinquency, 27
depersonalization, 48–9
Donne, John, cit., 10
double personality, 47

ego, the, 9
empathy, 7, 9–12, 17
    burial or cremation wishes and,
    11–12
    sex differences in formation of,
    10–11
Erikson, Erik, 3, 36

family, the, (families), 31
    Chinese, 26–7
    identification in, 29–30
'family romance', 44, 45, 49
Freud, Anna, 19, 43
friendship, 13–14

girls, dress of, 33
Greek mythology, 34

263

Index

group(s), 47, 48
  in- and out-, 19–20
  individuality and, 22–3
  membership and identity of,
    15–25
  reference, 20

hatred, identification and, 14–15
Healy, W., 47
home, 18
Hong-Kong, 24
humour, 17
Hutterites, 16
hysteria, 48

identification,
  child-parent, 12–13
  further aspects of, 25–30
  hatred and, 14–15
  individuals and, 25–9
  in families, 29–30
  with others, 12–15
identity,
  basic plot of, 40
  breakdown, 48–9
  breaks in, 36–7
  change, 21–2, 42
  continuity, coherence, and flex-
    ibility, 34–8
  definitions, 4
  development of, 5–9
  disturbances of, 48
  first approach to, 4–5
  formation of, 37–8, 45–8
  further cultural factors and, 30–3
  group membership and, 15–25
  hierarchy of, 37–8, 45–8
  organization of, 8–9
  reasons for choosing, 2–3
  social conventions permitting
    changes of, 45–6
  strength, 36, 37
  style of, 41–2
  unusual forms of, 42–4

incognito, 45
individualism, 23–5
individuality, group and, 22–3
individuals, identification of, 25–9
Israel, 44

Janet, P., 48

Kibbutzim, 44
Kluckhohn, C., 4
'Kwan Yin', 34

labels, 27–9
laughter, 16–18
leadership, 18–19
loss of memory, 4–5
'low-waist gang', 32

Manicheans, 16
mating, 13–14
mental health implications, 50
Metamorphoses, 49
migration, 43–4
morality, 20–1
multiple identities, 38
Murray, H. A., 4

names, 22, 27–9
nationalism, 33
Nazis, 19
Nirvana, 34
nom de plume, 45–6

operations, 46
Ovid, 49

petting, 32
Phaethon, 49
Philippines, 14, 21, 32
  rape in, 37
principle of positivism, 50
psycho-analysis, 35, 44
psychodrama, 21–2

Radcliffe-Brown, A. R., 5–6
reciprocity, 4
reincarnation, 24, 25, 35
Roth, Martin, 48
roots, 18

sainthood, 25
schizophrenia, 48
Scientific Committee, 2
sex, differences in empathy formation, 10–11
social role, 30–1
somatic sensitivity, 6–8
status, 30–1
strains, on identity, 37, 46
suttee, 47
symbiosis, 6

Teddy-boys, 32
transmigration of souls, 34–5
twins, identical, 5–6

U.S.A., the, 36
  names in, 28
  youth in, 32

WFMH, 2
'widgies and bodgies', 32
wit, 17

youth groups, 32

zoot-suiters, 32

Index

2. MENTAL HEALTH AND VALUE SYSTEMS

adaptation, 75–6, 109–10, 116, 229–30
'Good', The, and, 83–4
adolescence, 218
constructive use of, 217–18
adoption, Hindu, 142–3
Alexander, Franz, 102
analgesia, 160
Anglicanism, 135–6, 157–8
Anguttara Nikāya, cit., 78
anxiety, 140, 197
responsibility and, 187–8
anxiety state, history of cases of, 195–6
Assaad, Jalal el Din, 119
Authoritarian Personality, 223
authority, 233–4
'autism', 206
Avicenna, 208

babies, 113–14
'bad man', the, 82
balance, 114–15
Bali, 104
behaviour *see also* catatonic behaviour, psychotic behaviour
adaptive, 229–30
deviant, 88–104, 116
social attitudes to wrong, 93–4
belief,
mental health worker and, 180–1
patient's, 181–3
Bhagavadgita, cit., 79
Bowlby, J., 105
boys, values set on, 198–9
Brahminism, 81, 127–9, 136, 194
'brainwashing', 153, 185–6

Buddhism, 66, 77, 105–6, 175, 176, 177, 234

Calvinism, 151
Canada, 137, 138, 139
canonization, 103
caste system, 106–7, 133
catatonic behaviour, 102, 235
catharsis, 154
change, 173–4, 183, 202, 203, 204, 209, 228–9
Moslem concept of, 134–5
child, the, (children),
care of, 200–3
communication and, 215
development of, 96–7
experience of death of others and, 199
intuition in, 205–6
neglect of, 105
orientation and, 214–5
right and, 147–57, 226
wrong and, 147–57, 226
childbirth, 160
Chinese communism, 131, 153, 185
Chinese Emperors, 122
Christianity, 62, 67, 79–80, 97, 105–6, 222, 234
sexuality and, 151–2
suffering and, 157–9
circumcision, 89–90, 91
coercion, 184
communication, child and, 215
communism *see also* Chinese communism, 68
concern for others, 234
conformity, 84–6, 88–92, 111

Confucianism, 67, 83–4, 120–2, 132, 146, 166
  Marxism and, 131, 152–3
  responsibility of society and individual and, 126–7
  sexuality and, 150–1
  suffering and, 159
Confucius, cit., 78–9
Consensus of Opinion, 134–5
conversion, 154
conviction, definiteness of, 216–17
corporal punishment, 91
Corinthians, cit., 80
crime, 93–4
culpability, 94–6
culture(s), 65–6, 111, 112–13, 162, 183
  levels of aspiration in a, 235–6
  treatment and 177–80, 206–7

d'Arc, Jeanne, 103
death,
  children and, 199, 226
  different attitudes to, 157–62
delinquency, 129–30
dependence, independence and, 232–3
Deuteronomy, cit., 79
Dhammapada, on good, cit., 77
disintegration, 217
dream interpretation, 178
Dukhobors, 66

East, the, 170, 171
eccentrics, 98–100
ecstasy, 101–4
eidetic imagery, 102
emotional relationships, intensity of, 231
environmental change, 82–3
environmental determinism, 130–1
Erikson, Erik, 96–7
ethics, psychiatric treatment and, 183–7

Existentialism, 84

family, the, (families), 170, 200–3, 204
  Brahmin, 129
  change and, 174–16
  different patterns in life of, 146–7, 215–16
  Hindu, 141–3
  Islamic, 145
  Jewish, 67, 144–5
  monogamous, 152
  Nigerian, 145–6
  social relationships within, 105–6
  society and, 224
fanaticism, 236–7
fasting, history of a case of, 194–5
father, the, 146–7, 216
  Confucian attitude to, 144
filial piety, 145
First Asian Seminar on Mental Health and Family Life (Tsung-yi Lin, 1958), 170
flexibility, 132–40, 166–7
  tolerance and, 232
flying saucers, 102
France, 137, 138, 139
function, differentiation of, 224–5

girls, values set on, 198–9
God, 67, 121, 125
  belief in, 87–8
  Hindu, 132, 133
  mental illness and, 163, 164
Goethe, 132
'Good', The, social adaptation and, 83–4
'good man', the, 76–82
  Hindu view of the, 81–2
growth, 114–15, 228–9
guilt, 97, 148, 159
  different attitudes to, 157–62

hallucinations, 102, 103

Index

harmony, 86–7
happiness, 73
Hata Yogins, 123–4
Hazen Foundation, 61
health, defined by WHO, 70
Hebrew religion, 67, 79
    family and, 144–5
    flexibility of, 133–4
Hinduism, 81, 102, 132, 152, 166,
    194, 220
    boys and girls and, 198–9
    caste system of, 106–7
    death and suffering and, 161
    flexibility of, 132–3, 136–7
    holy man, the, of, 123–4
    individual responsibility within a
        collective system, 127–9
    joint family system of, 141–3
history, 122
holy man, 123–4
hospital admission, 184, 185
human development, 214–8
Hutterites, 66

identity, 131–2, 230–1
ideologies, relevant material from
    various, 118–68
illness, Chinese and Confucian atti-
    tude towards, 127
imagery, 124–5
influence of, 236
independence, 107–9
    dependence and, 232–3
India, 149–50, 161
    boys and girls in, 198
    change in, 175
    underprivileged in, 128–9
Indian students, 196
Indians, North American, 102
individual, the,
    involvement in religious practice
        of, 234–5
    society, responsibility and, 125–31

individual aspirations, community
    goals and, 219–20
insanity, 97, 103
instruction, efficacy of religious
    and ethical, 221
intellect, 207–8
International Congress on Mental
    Health (1948), 71
intuition, 205–6
    rapport and, 207–8
Islam, 62, 67–8, 73, 80, 88–9,
    119–20, 148–9, 152
    concept of change in, 134–5
    concept of utility in, 155–7
    veil in, 196
    women in, 177

Jains, the, 152
Judaism see Hebrew religion

Karma, 128
Khartoum, 156
Koran, the, 134, 152
    dream interpretation and, 178
Ku Klux Klan, 218

law, Islamic, 135
leucotomy, 186–7
liberty, 184–5
Lun Yu, cit., 78–9

Mafia, 218
Majjhima Nikāya, cit., 78
marriage(s), 107–12
    Hindu, 142
    mixed, 225–6
    problems, 189
Marxism, 68, 130, 131
    Confucianism and, 152–3
Matthew, cit., 80
maturity, 107–9, 228–9
'maturity at age', religious ideology
    and, 220

mendicants, 99, 100
mental health,
  aspirations and, 149–50
  concepts of, 65, 139
  defined by the International Congress on Mental Health, 71
  in changing societies, 110–11
  Islamic concept of, 119–20
  measurement of, 68–9
  nature of, 70–88
mental health practices, 223–7
mental health work, different ways of introducing, 173, 223–4
mental health worker, the, 180, 193–4, 209, 210, 239
  minister of religion and, 188–92
  role of, in the absence of specific value systems, 225
  specialization of functions of, 192–3
mental hospitals, 100–1
mental illness, 142
  attitudes towards, 162–4, 227
  Chinese and Confucian attitude towards, 127
minister of religion, the, mental health worker and, 188–92
missions, selection of personnel of religious, 223
Mogul invasions, 198
moral well-being, 73
Moslems *see* Islam
mother-child relationship, 105–6, 113–14, 115, 143–4, 177, 216
mysticism (mystics), 102, 163–4

Nazism, 84–5, 95
Negroes, American, 106
Neumann, Theresa, 103–4
neurosis, 81, 85, 109, 129, 130, 141, 142, 175
  among religious people, 222
  missionaries and, 223

Nigeria,
  death in, 162
  dual loyalties in, 197–8
  family in, 145–6
  society is the law, 129–30
Nigerian students (1951–4 study), 196
nutrition, 68–9

objective reality, 74
objectivity, 206–7
orientation, child and, 214–5

parental priestly role, 219
parental role, psychological treatment and, 219
parent figure, repudiation of wrong, and relationship with, 96–7
patient, the, respect for values of, 181–3, 225
Philippians, cit., 80
physical health, 65
polygamy, 119–20, 155, 156
prayer practices, 222
prevention, 172
principle of positivism, 230
'productive disintegration', 217
Psalms, cit., 79
psychiatric treatment, and ethics, 183
psychiatrist, the, Sudanese concept of, 192–3
psychological treatment, parental role and, 219
psychology, studies in, 218–23
psychoneurosis *see* neurosis
psychosis, among religious people, 223
psychotherapy, 154–5, 173, 186, 187, 193
psychotic behaviour, 100–1, 109
purdah, release from, 195–6

rapport, intuition and, 207–8

rationalization, 74
relationship(s),
    intensity of emotional, 200–3, 231
religion(s)   *see also* minister of
    religion
    individual and, 234–5
    neurosis and psychosis and, 222–3
    relevant material from various,
        118–68
    studies in psychology and,
        218–23
research, some leads into, 212–37
responsibility, 125–31, 233
    anxiety and, 187–8
Resurrection, the, 158–9
Revelation, 138
right, concepts of, 147–57, 226
rigidity, 218
ritual practices, analogies in com-
    pulsive behaviour and, 222
ritualism, compulsive, 221–2
Roman Catholicism, 95, 103, 137,
    138–9, 151, 158–9, 166, 187,
    188, 189
Rümke, 72
    on guilt, cit., 97
Russia *see* Soviet Russia (Union)

sadism, 91
Samoa, 108
Samyutta Nikāya, cit., 78
Scientific Committee, 61, 63
Senyussi, the, 99, 123
sexuality, attitudes to, 150–2
shame, 97, 148, 159
Shun, Emperor, 122
siblings, 146–7, 203
sikhism, 160
    attainable ideal of, 120
    death and suffering and, 161
social adaptation, 75–6
    'Good', The, and, 83–4
social conformity, 84–6, 88–92
social harmony, 86–7

social organization, 140–7
social relationships, 105–11
society, 74–5
    family and, 224
    Hinduism and individual position
        in, 128
    responsibility, individual and,
        125–31
Socrates, 102–3
Soddy, K., cit., 72
Soviet Russia (Union), 88
    attitude to error in, 152–3
    individual and, 130
    value systems in, 122
spiritual life, 209
storm troopers, 85–6
Sudan, the, 119–20, 135, 156, 157,
        178
    illness in, 162
    mystics in, 163–4
    psychiatrist in, 192–3
suffering,
    children and, 226
    different attitudes to, 157–62
    socially unacceptable behaviour
        and, 92–3
Surah, cit., 80–1
suttee, 198–9
sympathy, 206–7

Taoism, 66–7
toleration (tolerance),
    flexibility and, 232
    in society of deviant behaviour,
        97–101
tonsillectomy, 90–1
tragedy, 160
trances, 104
'twilight states', 102

U.S.A., the, 131
    attitudes to death in, 199
    Authoritarian Personality in, 223

Muslims in, 173–4
universal phenomena, 112–15
untouchables, 150–1
utility, Moslem concept of, 155–7

vagrants, 99
value systems, 119–25
values, forced acceptance of new, 203–4
    threat to central cultural, 183
veil, the, wearing, 196
virtue, 73

weaning, 115

West, the, 170, 171
WHO Constitution, 70
'whole man', the, concept of, 73
women, 178
    Hindu, 198–9
    Moslem world, 177
wrong, 93–4
    concepts of, 147–57, 226
    repudiation of, and relationship
    with parent figure, 96–7

Yao, Emperor, 122
Yoga *see also* Hata Yogins, 164–5

Printed and bound by CPI Group (UK) Ltd, Croydon, CR0 4YY

01/11/2024

01782632-0011